ON GETTING OFF

Damon Young is a prize-winning philosopher and writer. He is the author or editor of thirteen books, including *The Art of Reading*, *How to Think About Exercise*, *Philosophy in the Garden*, and *Distraction*. His works have been translated into eleven languages, and he has also written poetry, short fiction, and children's fiction. Young is an Associate in Philosophy at the University of Melbourne.

ON
GETTING
OFF

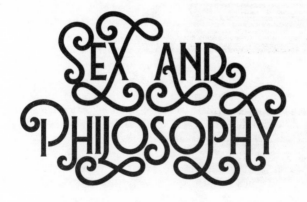

DAMON
YOUNG

SCRIBE
Melbourne • London

Scribe Publications
2 John St, Clerkenwell, London, WC1N 2ES, United Kingdom
18–20 Edward St, Brunswick, Victoria 3056, Australia
3754 Pleasant Ave, Suite 100, Minneapolis, Minnesota 55409, USA

Published in Australia and New Zealand by Scribe 2020
Published in the UK by Scribe 2021

Typeset in Sabon by the publishers
Printed and bound in the UK by CPI Group (UK) Ltd, Croydon CR0 4YY

Scribe Publications is committed to the sustainable use of natural resources
and the use of paper products made responsibly from those resources.

9781912854233 (UK edition)
9781925849219 (Australian edition)
9781950354559 (US edition)
9781925938555 (ebook)

Catalogue records for this book are available from the National Library
of Australia and the British Library.

scribepublications.co.uk
scribepublications.com.au
scribepublications.com

'... "explanation by sex" tends for us to
have a kind of intuitive obviousness, as if
we perfectly knew what sex was.'
IRIS MURDOCH
Metaphysics as a Guide to Morals

'How many things are possible, in the
immense universe of Heaven and Earth!'
PU SONGLING
'The Fornicating Dog'

CONTENTS

The Classroom

On the Sudden Strangeness of Sex

I will begin where this began for me: A's legs.

It was the late eighties, in a portable classroom. Black aluminium window frames, laminated tables with rounded edges, a wonky dark green blackboard. Summer stuffiness. Perhaps the teacher — thick-rimmed glasses, high belted trousers, chronic sneer — was speaking. Perhaps not. The lesson did not matter.

I was looking at a classmate.

A had her knees up on the desk, and was rocking back and forth. It was enthralling. Or, more correctly: I was enthralled.

I had seen legs before — alongside bellies and backs and chests. In first grade, one fellow pupil even pulled her underwear down. I did the same. But this was hilarious, not arousing. As a young child, bodies were occasionally a joke, mostly unseen and unexciting.

A's legs, they were suddenly very visible to me — and not funny at all. They felt like an invitation. They were not, of course. A was oblivious to my existence. And I later realised my own obliviousness, casually turning another human being into a prop for my pleasure. But honesty is important here: it *felt* like her skin was there for me; was an offering.

An offering of what? There were not yet even vague fantasies. For all my illusions of invitation, there was no address on the envelope; no party to attend. I had longing, but not for anything. This was pure yearning. It is awkward to use the word 'desire' about a child: it seems anachronistic and crude. But the word does justice to my memories. I was eleven years old, and feeling the beginnings of arousal; the buds of lust.

Plaited and Puzzling

It was a strange sensation. It felt familiar, this need. It was part of a well-known world: the same uniforms and accents, chalkdust and pencil sharpenings. I was myself, surely. Yet this was totally new: novel enough for me to remember it, decades later. Nothing in my childhood made sense of this. I had urges for lasagne or toy robots, but I wanted to eat or play with these; they had some obvious use. A wasn't *for* anything. She was just there: someone I had to look at, because the mere existence of her calves and thighs gave me a gut ache. A pleasant gut ache.

This 'had to look' was also weird: I felt pushed into gazing. The urge felt profoundly intimate, like no one else would or could feel this way. And these are straightforwardly my memories — or my memories of memories, at least. They have a first-person mineness to them; an atmosphere of selfhood. Yet the nudge was not wholly mine. It felt automatic: a necessity of feeling, if not of behaviour. In short, it was not quite my arousal. It was like the hand of a stranger on the back of my skull. Look, it shoved. *Look*.

This, in turn, meant that I was no longer wholly Damon. For the first time, I felt at odds with myself. No other basic needs had done this, perhaps because they arose in infancy, and were soon part of my growing psyche. As a school-aged child, I never felt undone by or uncomfortable about hunger, thirst, or the dash for the toilet. But this? It was like I had been invaded, and this alien had made itself at home in me — *as* me.

What had changed? A was the same, with the same goody-two-shoes demeanour. I was the one transformed: this odd longing, rising up within me. Yet it felt like the world had shifted too; like its meniscus had a new sheen. A's legs suddenly had charm. This charisma spread across her whole persona, making her someone I wanted to know. (This never happened. The want was enough.) This had a curious physicality to it. I did not merely feel A was sexy — she *was* sexy. There was no naysaying this new reality. Put another way, my lust was now part of the universe. It was as much a fact as the smell of the canteen's sausage rolls or teacher's cigarettes.

Alongside this fact was lack. Gaping in the classroom, I felt I was missing something. I was simply not enough on my own. I needed A. Or, a little later, her friend B. Or my neighbour, C. Or him, or her, or they, or, or ... This need sacrificed the present on the altar of the future, offering more in fantasy than reality provided. It was distracting. This was the beginning of a lifetime's deficit. Not because I needed some romantic union, some eternal gathering of selves. The dearth was erotic, and no one person could meet it. Looking back, I doubt it can be met. For me, desire is restless and seemingly endless, and what changes is its force not its logic. It is often foolish.

As a child, I had been warned about adolescence: the chuckled warnings, the medical explanations. The portrait was chiefly physiological, full of hair, bumps and tumescence. This was all true and sometimes awkward. But no one nodded to the existential trauma of sexuality; the way the cosmos and I seemed to split apart. It was familiar but shocking; mine but foreign; within me but 'out there'; promising some ultimate satisfaction, but offering little but want.

I also recognised — eventually, embarrassingly — my denial of A's selfhood; the way she became legs first, and a person very distantly second — if at all. She, and countless others. I was a somewhat alienated child, curious about others' selves. I laboured to understand, and still do. But with A, I gave up — and did so happily. My desire for her was far greater than my desire to know her. Put simply: I became an objectifier in that classroom, turning a subject into a thing for my jollies.

Much later, I felt a double gaze: my lover like a mere thing for me, and I for them — yet both of us still full selves. I learned about the 'tender indignities' of fucking, as Frank Herbert put it in *Dune*.

In all of this, sex was an invitation to philosophy. Since the beginnings of thought, humanity has been challenged and provoked by schisms. The sudden observation that things were not what they seemed; that ancient customs were fragile or relative; that language and know-how were often at odds; that solving riddles often led to new riddles — that, in short, the universe was no longer a commonsense thing: this was a prompt for thinkers. And every generation added new questions to the answers. Sages, boffins, gadflies — each confronted a cosmos full of holes, folds and rips.

As the French philosopher Maurice Merleau-Ponty observed, intimacy is an experience of exactly this sort. Not because it affords sacred epiphanies or biological certainties, but because its sensations and perceptions are so equivocal. They resist easy summary into flesh or mind, you or me, inside or outside, fact or value, and so on. 'We never know whether the forces which bear us on are [the body's] or ours,' Merleau-Ponty noted in *The Phenomenology of Perception*, 'or with the result rather that they are never entirely its or ours.' To fuck, or to want to fuck, or to have the first lurch or leaning towards this want? This is to feel our basic human ambiguity.

So existence is plaited and puzzling, and sex highlights this — sometimes beautifully, sometimes grotesquely.

It Comes in Threes

What do I mean by 'sex'? Following philosopher Irving Singer, I think of sex as 'libido', 'eros', and 'romance'. Each of these is a kind of basic need — and none are more basic than the other.

The libidinal is about getting our rocks off. Singer describes the libido as 'a somewhat automatic trigger for generating behavioral and physiological processes related to reproduction'. It is not necessarily about making babies, but it does involve fundamental biological urges, reflexes and cycles. For all our psychological and social subtleties, this is *Homo sapiens*' equivalent to rutting. It involves the kind of mania celebrated in DH Lawrence's *Lady Chatterley's Lover* ('short and sharp, he took her, short and sharp and finished, like an animal') and parodied in Phillip Roth's *Portnoy's Complaint* ('when I was fifteen I took it out of my pants and whacked off on the 107 bus').

The erotic is the aesthetic joy we take in others, and which I took in A's legs. Singer calls the erotic 'the affective glue that binds us to other persons, things, or ideals, and to ourselves'. This is Sophia in Deborah Levy's *Hot Milk*, revelling in her new lover Ingrid. 'I like … the way she takes off her heavily embroidered belt … how her bare feet are covered in red dust … the way she says my name in English'. Importantly, and as Levy's Sophia suggests, eros need not be visual. It might be the feel of goosebumps on someone's thigh, the swagger in their walk, the rasp of their voice. Marlon James' novel *Black Leopard, Red Wolf* is thick with scents, including the second smell of a man: 'one that hides under the arms, between the legs, between the buttocks, what you smell when close enough to touch with lips'.

Eros need not be libidinal either. As feminist author Shulamith Firestone noted in *The Dialectic of Sex*, we can respond erotically to various and varied others — from lovers to friends. It is not just a genital swelling, but a 'spark', as she puts it, which fires over 'the spectrum of our lives'. Because of this, we can have a broadly erotic response to objects other than human beings. In *Watermark*, Russian-born poet Joseph Brodsky wrote of the thrill of a gondola ride in Venice: 'the noiseless and traceless passage of its lithe body upon the water — much like sliding your palm down the smooth skin of your beloved'. Even without Brodsky's comparison, this is classic eros.

The romantic is about recognition: here is another human being, whose existence matters to me, and to whom I matter. It is what I strive for with Ruth, my wife. This is not some grand metaphysical union; the mixing of selves in Venus' grinder. Instead, it is about maintaining twoness: the commitment by lovers to one another's uniqueness. In Jeanette Winterson's *Oranges Are Not the Only Fruit*, Jeanette loves Katy for her brazen but sincere passion. They screw easily and happily, then Katy watches Jeanette at the pulpit. It is neither eternal love nor orthodox marriage, but it is real and good, and has to do with these very specific young women in very specific circumstances. Think also of the anonymous, invented lover in Alice Tarbuck's poem 'Mary Godwin Shelley's Second Wife'. She licks Mary while proclaiming feminist principles; she nurses her wife through loss and betrayal; she encourages confidence and laughter. She 'excises doubt/ and undoes clothes like a pocket knife,/ open at the blade.' This is carnal pleasure, yes — and rightly so. Yet it is also two beings addressed to one another. In romance, 'we are impelled toward persons,' Singer writes, 'who matter to us as the particularities we take them to be'. This does not mean we must care about our paramours forever, or that love equals monogamy. It does not mean we must only love one, rather than two or more. Instead, it simply means that we seek to care for this person, *as* this person — not as some flattering caricature, decoration, or entertainment. Our romance can be serial or simultaneous, for a life or for a summer.

The libidinal, erotic and romantic need not come together in one lover. We can fuck without devotion, adore without horniness, gape without love — this has been the stuff of literature and song, for millennia. Sex is neither purely mating nor purely doting, because it is purely nothing. It is a complex of lust, perception and care, which includes all the subtlety and caprice our odd species can offer.

And as Brodsky's gondola ride suggests, these cannot always be contained within sex itself — our lusts and loves can mingle in resonance, if not in fact. We can find ourselves in a shocking melange of intimacies. Witness Monica in Zadie Smith's short story 'Sentimental Education', who sleeps with three people in twelve hours, while at university. Decades later, she finds a 'faint echo' of this in breastfeeding her baby, nursing her older kid to sleep, then joining her partner in bed ('pressing backwards into the beloved, to nullify his flesh in hers, and vice versa'). Sex is part of life, and so even 'just fucking' is not always just fucking; its filaments reach widely.

Crime Against Life

So, sex is a tangle of libido, eros, and romance — and its tensions prompt philosophy. Or ought to. Yet sex talk is oddly superficial.

We are told that lust is a universal mania. The popular impression is of a civilisation of Priapuses or Aphrodites, throbbing from fantasy to fantasy. And much of daily life is certainly sexualised, if not sexual: typically while trying to sell us something. We are supposedly always thinking about sex. But what exactly is a 'thought' here? A conscious notion, a fugitive impression, a lingering mood? The measures are often vague at best. And much of the research that finds hundreds or thousands of horny thoughts seems biased: asking about the libido primes the libido, or gender stereotypes guide estimates. Psychologist Terri Fisher and colleagues, writing in the *Journal of Sex Research*, conclude that most of these studies have had 'weak' methodologies. Their own study reports fewer than nineteen sex thoughts a day for men, and ten for women.

And even if we are thinking about sex more often, we do not necessarily *think* about sex — not seriously. The thoughts just happen; they arise and fall away. Put another way, sex is often psychologically but not intellectually compelling.

Ironically, this is partly because desire matters so much. It puts cognition on hold, because we skip questions of 'what' or 'why' in favour of 'when'; the answers are practical, not meditative.

More importantly, we often value sex *as* this dumb fun or safe savagery. It becomes pure skin to skin, or beastliness, or loss of self in the other. In her memoir *The Sexual Life of Catherine M.*, writer and critic Catherine Millet remembers the beautiful anonymity of orgies; the free abandonment of herself to men. She does not know what she will be asked to do, or with whom. But she devotes herself single-mindedly to the sexual adventure. 'I feel more like a driver who must stick to the rails than a guide who knows where the port is,' she says of her career. 'I've fucked in the same way.' Similarly, theorist David Halperin describes gay bathhouses as opportunities for sex without elaborate straight courting rites. For him, one of the pleasures of the baths is being nothing but desirable flesh. '... you can, in total security,' he writes in 'What is Sex For?', 'aspire to be objectified, to be treated like a thing'. A tryst with others or oneself can feel like a way to shrug off the anxieties and exhaustions of daily life. We find what James Baldwin, in his novel *Another Country*, called 'the flaming torpor of passivity'.

Many moralists agree that sex is brute or dumb in this way, but think it is dangerous for this very reason. For them, we do not merely use sex to avoid thinking — screwing *is* this avoidance. Lust becomes a fiend that somehow strips us of reason and freedom.

European philosophers and theologians have been at the forefront of this campaign against carnal joy. These patriarchs have deemed lust ignoble or simply ignored it altogether.

Witness Plato's hand-wringing in the fourth century before Christ. The Athenian is widely regarded as one of the grandfathers of Western thought. And rightly so: his writings are beautiful, provocative, and sometimes moving.

As with so many of our origins, Plato's dialogues are deceptively familiar. It is easy to look past what is bizarre about them. Especially as the author is so frank about lust. Like many Greeks of his era, he was raised without Christian shame. If he later pushed back against this idea, he still carried himself with a pagan straightforwardness. Witness his *Symposium*, which portrays flirting with wit and charm, and has no qualms about describing Alcibiades' erect persona. As philosopher Alfred North Whitehead noted, this is one of the marks of Plato's genius: not simply the Athenian's ideas, but his talent for putting those ideas in their rich psychological and social surroundings. Plato 'provides his own environing sociological interpretation,' as Whitehead once put it in conversation.

What strikes me in his interpretation is that sex is a problem. Not this rimjob or that pegging, but sex *per se*. It is not simply one part of a good life, which must be negotiated cannily. It is an enemy of the good life — that is, an enemy of philosophy. It might briefly be an ally, but it can never be trusted. Better to do away with it altogether.

Yes, Plato himself was brilliant, handsome, muscular and wealthy — often the hallmarks of a life dedicated to worldly pleasures. And he was no virgin. Yet his works describe the flesh as a prison or heavy weight, which keeps good citizens from escaping or ascending to truth. Love is healthy — it invites us to the Good itself. In fact, even lust for a handsome boy is healthy, as long as it orients the lover towards goodness. But Plato believed celibacy is the best lifestyle, promoting 'self-mastery and inward peace'.

He provided a dramatic emblem for this outlook, which also characterises so much later thought. In his *Republic*, he depicted a conversation with the poet Sophocles, then an old man. Someone asks the playwright if he still pays 'service to Aphrodite'. A very civilised way of wondering if he still likes to fuck. Sophocles' reply is famous: 'Hush, man, most gladly have I escaped this thing you talk of, as if I had run away from a raging and savage beast of a master.' For Plato, my classroom epiphany was the moment this master began to fetter me.

A generation after Plato, the early Stoics were not prudish about sex. Chrysippus praised Diogenes the Cynic for wanking publicly, while Zeno recommended swinging. But each of these ideas arose from a greater fear of commitment: wanking in front of others supposedly makes us less in thrall to the crowd; sharing lovers less in the thrall of any one. In the later Stoics, this fear seemed to grow stronger. Ever the cold fish, Epictetus described succumbing to passion as a 'defeat'. Even the worldly statesman Seneca called desire a 'secret destruction'. (He was writing to Helvia, his grieving mother. As one does.) This alarm at passion was typical of a philosophy obsessed with mental ease. Third-century historian Diogenes Laërtius summed up Stoicism's flight in this way: 'to be in transports of delight is the melting away of virtue.'

The word 'Epicurean' suggests excess nowadays, but Epicurus himself was austere. The philosopher and commune leader believed that sex was natural but superfluous. Laërtius paraphrased him in this way: 'No one was ever the better for sexual indulgence, and it is well if he be not the worse.' Like most Greeks and Romans, the Epicureans were not naive about sexuality. They recognised that it was often healthier to relieve lust than not, especially if longing led to pain. In his philosophical poem *On the Nature of Things*, written at least a century after Epicurus died, Lucretius was typically practical. It is better, he wrote, 'to cast the collected liquid into any body, and not to retain it,' than to chase a beloved. Put another way: fucking just anyone is safer than loving a bedmate. The ideal, of course, was to avoid sex altogether, doing away with the mere chance of suffering. Passion was a threat to *ataraxia*: equanimity.

The third-century Roman philosopher Plotinus was no virginal naïf, once seemingly using penetration as a metaphor for union with the divine. 'A kind of passionate experience like that of a lover,' he wrote in his *Enneads*, 'resting in the beloved.' Despite his concerns about 'blood or menstrual discharges', he was also no stranger to physical beauty. But as a typical Platonist, he was wary of actual sex — figurative fucking was more godly than literal. In his grand metaphysical hierarchy, rising from the material depths to the ethereal heights was best achieved with chastity. He seemed tolerant in life, many of his students marrying and having children. But his theory was clear: desire is healthy, if what we desire is the ultimate ideal. This is how oneness is achieved, not with dross stuff; not merely with the coupling of organs. 'It is error,' he pronounced, 'to fall away into sexual intercourse.' His biographer, fellow Neoplatonist Porphyry, wrote that Plotinus was 'ashamed of being in the body'.

Speaking of loathing for the flesh: to Christianity. Plotinus and other Platonists were strong influences on the fourth- and fifth-century theologian Augustine of Hippo. As a youth, Augustine seemingly slept with many lovers, and invented others to impress his mates. But after an ill-fated affair with an older woman (who bore him a child), the North African scholar converted to Christianity and rounded on lust. His morality was ethereal, believing we had to die in this world to live in God's. He saw carnality as dangerous, wrenching our spirits back to profane existence. For Augustine, our genitals are willful and capricious, and procreation without orgasm is the ideal. In his Paradise, men ejaculate like they might reach for a fruit: calmly, with no shudder. This is, he wrote in *Against Julian*, 'the movement of peaceful will by which we command the other members of the body'. The virtuous soul will not be ruled by flesh, even as he spills his seed.

Aristotle rarely discussed sex and sexuality, but his outlook guided scholarship in Europe and the Near East during the middle ages — for many centuries, he was known as simply 'the Philosopher'. Thirteenth century theologian Thomas Aquinas married Augustine's fear of lust to Aristotle's virtue theory, and idea of a purposeful universe. Their offspring was the ideal of a mildly contented breeder. For Aquinas, we were not made by

God to wank or suck one another. These are all sins. The only allowable fucking is between a married man and woman, and makes babies (or tries to). 'The use of venereal acts can be without sin,' he wrote, 'provided they be performed in due manner and order, in keeping with the end of human procreation.' Like the Philosopher, Aquinas argued all this very calmly; the pages of his *Summa Theologica* lack Augustine's stink of brimstone. And he was not against carnal joy, yoked by the firm hands of reason. Still, his overall conception of sexual pleasure was typically philosophical. As John Milhaven notes in his essay 'Thomas Aquinas and Sexual Pleasure', Aquinas saw lust as stupid. We cannot learn anything while screwing worthy of the name 'knowledge'. 'Lust gives rise to blindness of mind,' he warned, 'which excludes almost entirely the knowledge of spiritual things'.

In the fifteenth century, Marsilio Ficino was the founder and head of the Academy in Florence, named after Plato's school. He translated Plato into Latin and Italian, and is credited with the still-used phrase 'Platonic love'. Ficino was no stranger to Aristotelian and Scholastic ideas, but he made Plato's erotic yearning the heart of his philosophy. Very much a Renaissance Christian, he saw love of beauty as a way to salvation. We begin with perhaps a noble profile and a supple calf, and end with atonement. Importantly, he meant hot guys — ladies were just for babies. (In German, *florenzen*: to sodomise.) Yet for all his erotic metaphors, Ficino treated fucking itself with tolerance at best, contempt at worst. He caviled against those who do 'disgraceful things' like anal intercourse, foolishly believing that 'only by ejaculating or recieving this, they can surrender or receive the whole body.' Ficino was right that penetration need not lead to transcendent union. But for the wrong reasons. He clearly loved the younger Giovanni Cavalcanti, but was wary of 'the filths of the body', as he put it in *De Amore*. This outlook was common to many of his followers and fellow Neoplatonists: screwing is safer as an intellectual or poetic trope than as an actual part of philosophical life.

On sex, the most radical departure from medieval and Renaissance ideas came in the eighteenth century. With their confident materialism, *philosophes* like Jean-Jacques Rousseau, Denis Diderot and Voltaire did away with many shibboleths about unnatural and unhealthy practices. Diderot, for example, wrote a fictional dialogue in 1769 that praised masturbation. He had the French doctor and *Encyclopédiste* Théophile de Bordeu recommending wanking to his younger friend, the salon host Mademoiselle de L'Espinasse. It felt marvellous, eased stress, and avoided madness, allowing 'the superabundant humour' to be relieved. This was not Bordeu's public prescription — as with homosexuality, he knew better than to support so-called 'crimes' against French society. But privately, he suggested that celibacy was a greater threat to happiness and well-being than a good rub. 'We must never force nature,' the physician continued, 'but we can give her a helping hand when need arises.'

The Marquis de Sade took this brazen materialism and turned it against his era's genteel rationality. Like the *philosophes*, he believed that a physical universe liberated us from the morality of religious authorities. But Sade went further, claiming that there was no morality whatsoever. There was just Nature. 'Had Nature condemned sodomy's pleasures, incestuous correspondences, pollutions, and so forth,' he asked in his 1795 *Philosophy in the Bedroom*, 'would she have allowed us to find so much delight in them?' Yet Nature is also random and literally careless, so we follow her only in capricious destruction. Philosopher Timo Airaksinen sums up Sade's seemingly adolescent maxim: 'Whatever principles exist must be broken.' No mere theorist, the aristocratic aesthete used his position to rape and torture the poor, eventually being jailed then committed for his crimes. For all his supposed rebellion, the Marquis was typical. Yet another powerful man abusing women. And yet another thinker who made sense of sex only by stripping it of everything but pure physicality — in this, he was a philosopher's philosopher.

Despite the enormous mark left by many of these Enlightenment thinkers, their celebrations of sex did little for philosophy more generally, especially into the next century. Their playful — and sometimes necessarily private — discussions were not the stuff of 'serious' scholarship. David Hume wrote of lust with typically commonsense care in *A Treatise of Human Nature*, but only briefly. Meanwhile, the world-conquering Germans of the eighteenth and nineteenth centuries, Immanuel Kant and George Wilhelm Friedrich Hegel, were both frustratingly conservative about screwing: fucking is allowable in marriage. (As far as we know, Kant was a virgin. Hegel fathered an illegitimate child.)

A notable exception to this tight-lipped orthodoxy was Arthur Schopenhauer, who was candid about the power of lust — and worried for this very same reason. He argued that all life is driven by the Will: pure, restless becoming. This force takes hold of us, directing us to make babies. We screw, not for ourselves, but for this brute and stupid Will behind all organisms. Putting aside the question of whether or not Schopenhauer was right, what is most striking about his philosophy is his contempt for lust. He did not want to celebrate sex. He called it 'a malevolent demon who is trying to pervert, confuse, and overthrow everything'. He wanted to do away with the demon, along with all longings. His vision of the ultimate life was one of numbed tranquility. (He failed to achieve this.)

These thinkers cannot sum up even European philosophy. Plato was once called an 'alien drop' in the Greek bloodstream, and many of these men were Platonists of a stripe: Plotinus, Augustine, Ficino, Schopenhauer. And they were all *men*: philosophy was an ancient game of tug-of-war between phalluses. As philosophers Fiona Jenkins and Katrina Hutchinson observe, my vocation has 'actively and systematically disparaged women's very capacity for its key qualifying attribute — the possession of reason itself.' I suspect it still does.

But as extremes, these men are surprisingly representative of a long line of pearl-clutching scholars. In the work of so many otherwise-reasonable thinkers, sex was either avoided altogether as silly or trivial, tolerated as domestic procreation, or condemned as vulgar. Not until Friedrich Nietzsche, who died at the beginning of the twentieth century, do we find an epochal philosopher actually celebrating the libido enthusiastically. 'Every expression of contempt for the sexual life,' he wrote in *Ecce Homo*, '… is *the* crime against life'. After a brief flirtation in the eighteenth century, only in the last century or so do we find philosophers really getting intimate with fucking. It took over two thousand years to get from Plato to what philosopher Alan Soble, in 'A History of Erotic Philosophy', calls 'an outpouring of sometimes shocking inquiries'.

In this, philosophy has historically been the meek cousin of debauchery. The grand libertine hurls himself into vacuity; the thinker runs away. Both often treat sex as something a bit stupid, and I want to correct this mistake. I echo the Scottish biographer and rake James Boswell, from his 1778 essay 'On Love': 'It is curious to consider philosophically the nature and effects of that passion, which, while a man is under its influence, deprives him of all philosophy.'

The Pleasure of Thought

So, sex rewards thought, but European philosophers have typically trivialised it. My intention here is to celebrate sex's intellectual suggestiveness; its power to coax a little philosophy from the little death. Thoughtless fucking is fun — but so is thinking about it.

If this seems odd, it is chiefly because scholars are stereotyped as numbed calculators, putting aside passion for thought. This cliché falsifies actual learning. As David Hume argued in his *A Treatise of Human Nature*, much boffinry is actually motivated by pleasure. '[O]f all other exercises of the mind,' Hume wrote, 'to fix our attention or exert our genius … is the most pleasant and agreeable.' The mind is like a muscle, and flexing it can be enjoyable. Strength, swiftness, finesse — each applies to minds as much as thews.

This does not mean that truth-seeking can be reduced to thrill-seeking; that facts or logic are merely entertainments. This muddles two kinds of ends: conclusions, and the rewards we get from pursuing them. It matters whether we think well or poorly; whether we are profound or shallow in our logic, careful or cavalier with facts. Hume's point is simply that anaesthetised duty is a caricature of scholarship. We get a buzz out of thinking, and this can be everything from a gentle contentment to a quivering thrill. These pleasures ought to be recognised alongside those of screwing or gazing at others screwing.

Importantly, Hume's theory does not say that pleasures are 'high' and 'low'; that intercourse is bestial whereas thinking about it is angelic. This often comes with a thoroughgoing dualism, dividing us into the carnal and the spiritual — and here we are back to Plato and his intellectual descendants. Physiologically speaking, gratification is gratification is gratification. In a paper for *Neuroethics*, philosopher Roger Crisp and neuroscientist Morten Kringelbach argue that our brains use the same kinds of connections and chemistry for orgies as they do for symposiums. And this makes evolutionary sense: successful species usually make do with what they have, rather than inventing new tissue, organs, neurotransmitters. So our pleasures have evolved, but not the mechanisms behind them. 'Pleasures of food, sex, addictive drugs, friends and loved ones, music, art,' they write, '… can produce strikingly similar patterns of brain activity.' Put simply: all joys ultimately involve the flesh.

So, reflecting on sex is enjoyable because reflecting is something bodies do — and bodies are made of receptive, responsive stuff. There is no otherworldly ether of ideas: we think through the same flesh we fuck with.

A Questioning Tone

But *how* to think about sex?

My form here is essayistic: my temperament is part of the work, and I am led by partial and very personal curiosity. As Martha Nussbaum argues in *The Fragility of Goodness*, philosophy best begins *within* life. It is 'fatal to accept this demand for an Archimedean point and for a pure, uninterpretive, translucent art of writing', she says. Perhaps the most absurd bias is the belief that we can be free of bias. Much of our life is reflex, habit, custom; much is value, even if this value is an interest in facts. Better to show my leanings than to disguise them.

Importantly, this essay form is not a permission slip for egotistical rambling. In 'The Decay of Essay-Writing', Virginia Woolf lamented 'the amiable garrulity of the tea-table', which cursed so many popular essays. Sex deserves diverse expertise: from philosophy and history, to psychology and biology. Still, there is no escaping the personality behind the scholarship. Woolf was wrong to believe that an essay must be wholly enchanting ('we must never be roused'), but right that it begins with some fixation or obsession — an 'obstinate conviction', as she put it in 'The Modern Essay'. Here, I look with obstinate conviction to notable sexual scenes for their tensions, frictions, contradictions; I find these in others, and in myself.

Writing about my own lust or fucking has not been simple. Most obviously, this is because sex so often makes for clumsy or cringeworthy prose. I take seriously historian Jacques Barzun's warning: that explicit descriptions are often more a political achievement than a literary one. They show that we are free to write what we please, not that we can write *well*. 'The single kiss in *The Golden Bowl* suffices *with the rest* to establish the intense sexuality of that novel,' Barzun wrote in 'Venus at Large', 'whereas many a modern work that might qualify as *coitus uninterruptus* is frigid.' I have not blushed to offer physical descriptions, but I have tried to give them a vivid or subtle humanity; to make them significant rather than simply shocking or uneasy — except when shock or uneasiness *is* the significance.

In discussing my own sex life, I have also negotiated the ethics of a common existence. My memories are certainly mine, with all the idiosyncrasy this suggests. But they involve others, and others at their most intimate. It is one thing to ask candour of myself — quite another to force this upon friends or lovers, by using them as cameos in my confessions.

Anyone recognisable in these pages has read these pages. Like the best screwing, this book arose from trust. None of us have enjoyed the final word, for there is no final word in literature. As Jean-Paul Sartre put it: 'One does not write for slaves.' I have used my freedom to invite theirs — and yours.

My experiences are limited, though — they are personally but not statistically significant. Alongside biographies and memoirs, I turn to novels, short stories, and poetry. This is partly because introducing others to good literature is one of the subtle joys of civilised life. Audre Lorde rightly described sharing as 'erotic' in her *Sister Outsider*. It offers understanding, yes. But it also allows others' quickened experience to enhance and enrich our own. Witness novelist (and bookshop owner) Ann Patchett on reading as adventure: 'When we stumble out again, like Shackleton from the Pole or Darwin off the Beagle, there is a tremendous desire to grab the first person we bump into and say, "Let me tell you what I've seen."' I claim this exploratory pleasure here.

But these literary references also have lasting intellectual value. They help to do justice to the diverse world of sexuality. It matters little that they are fictional; that Eric never really fucked Vivaldo in late fifties New York, because neither man in *Another Country* actually existed. What matters is that James Baldwin's novel expresses recognisably erotic, romantic, and libidinal ideas — and the worlds behind these ideas. In other words: it adds to our experience of things.

As John Dewey argued, life is essentially experience: an ambiguous to-and-fro between self and cosmos, animal and habitat, giving and receiving, doing and having-done-to.

Literature takes this vague and transient reality and makes it whole and still; turns experience into *an* experience. 'Tangled scenes of life are made more intelligible,' Dewey wrote in *Art as Experience*, '... by presenting their meanings as the matter of a clarified, coherent, and intensified ... experience.' While these tangled scenes are not originally our own, they enter into our consciousness. Importantly, this new intelligibility is not false simplicity. One of good literature's virtues is that it avoids falsifying reality, by making it too neat or conclusive. It offers many competing versions of life, and will not declare a winner. This is what philosopher Stuart Hampshire called 'an escape from security ... a certain kind of confusion'. Oftentimes art is most realistic when it abets this escape from certainty.

Art also bears witness to our escape *into* certainty: fantasy. Much of our sexual life is devoted to soothing possibilities; to 'if only', and 'perhaps', and 'maybe'. We are always half in a universe of consoling make-believe. 'The psyche is a historically determined individual relentlessly looking after itself,' wrote Iris Murdoch in 'The Sovereignty of Good Over Other Concepts'. 'One of its main pastimes is daydreaming.' Literature allows us to better see these illusions; to look them in the face, rather than squinting or gazing elsewhere for shame.

So, decades after I daydreamed about A's legs, I want to look more carefully at the new world they heralded. If we are divided creatures, I am curious about our navigation of this cleavage. Which sides do we cling to, or push away? What parts of ourselves do we laud or vilify, illuminate or darken, deem gorgeous or loathsome? Which cuts do we mend or widen?

Witness the questioning tone: I want sex to be the beginning, not the end, of a conversation.

A Warning

Sex and Trauma

I want to warn you, but also I do not want to warn you.

To begin: this is not a work of trauma. The atmosphere is often earnest, yes — but this is the earnestness of serious play, not of damage. So, a warning might introduce this book falsely; might prime you for terror or sadness that never arises.

But it is better to be prepared than shocked. Because sex so often involves others, it is ethical: there is scope for virtue and vice. Because sex happens within history, it is political: there is scope for oppression or emancipation, exclusion or inclusion, vilification or recognition. Sex can be vicious. Sex can be alienated. Sex can be just bad, where this 'bad' is not mere accident, but part of a logic of entitlement. Even at its most beautiful, fucking can involve brutality, violation, and a shuddering loss of self.

Yes, sex can offer some peace. But this 'can' avoids the enormous harm done by the lustful — including by those who lust for power.

In these pages, I discuss sex with candour; often with cheery enthusiasm. Yet I recognise that my delight might be your anxiety. Because this is how trauma works.

The word 'trauma' comes from the Greek for wound, and rightly so. When seriously traumatised, we are maimed. We lose vigour and suppleness. Our mental lacerations or lesions can become 'rationally eclipsing,' as philosopher Kate Manne puts it. The same damned causes keep having the same damned effects — hence that clumsy popular word, 'triggering'. This is partly why trauma is so grievous: it seems to turn us from rational agents into machines.

Philosophically, this mechanical trope is misguided and misleading. We are neither robots nor just reflexes. We have a sphere of liberty. And part of living with trauma is freely using our moments of poise and fortitude to cultivate ourselves. Survivors of trauma regularly confront what frightens us. Not out of bravado or masochism, but because this is how we exercise freedom; how we become more than what we are.

Still, I know what it is to feel primed; to feel like a jolt or spark is enough to ignite me. To this end, I have listed some of the more incendiary topics in this book. This is not because I condescendingly take responsibility for anyone's therapy, but because I *do not*: I defer to your liberty and judgement. I offer this information, trusting you will know what to do with it.

To change metaphors yet again, this warning is not a stop sign. It is a map. I am showing you where much of the difficult terrain lies. The territory is yours to explore.

Clowns: bestiality, transphobia.

Tiresias' Secret: pedophilia.

Choke Me: rape, violent sex.

Solomon Kane's Demon: misogyny and racism.
Fuckzilla: violent sex.
Solidarity: misogyny, rape, transphobia.
Akiko's Boys: rape, torture, pedophilia.
Prince and Lady: rape, misogyny, violent sex.

The Vulgar, Not the Vulgate

On Often Avoiding the Word 'Sex'

A brief note on the word, 'sex'. I find myself avoiding it often.

It is an ugly word. Not because it is boorish, but because it is too refined. 'Sex' is clinical: sterile, precise, institutional. It comes from the Norman French, originally Latin — what philologists Reneé and Henry Kahane called 'the status symbol of the rich, the powerful, the refined, and the snobbish'. It is the word of aristocratic victors, looking down upon Anglo-Saxon oiks.

Even today, 'sex' belongs in the official lexicon of government, business and academia. Adults use it in treatises and memoranda, often without sniggers or twitches. It is acceptable — that is to say, safe.

It is also very modern. For most of its history, 'sex' meant the division of the species into male and female. When Henry James, in *Portrait of a Lady*, wrote that Isabel Archer had the 'common genius of her sex', he was not referring to her boudoir gymnastics. He meant she was manipulative without guilt. (More proof that novelists can invent humans without always understanding humanity.) 'Sex' also meant genitals, a connotation that lasted at least three centuries from the seventeenth to the twentieth. A generation after Henry James, we finally see the newer sense in print: something you did or had. In his 1900 *Love and Mr Lewisham*, HG Wells quoted an orator saying 'we marry in fear and trembling, sex for a home is the woman's traffic'. The patriarchal exchange is old, alas — but the phrasing is new. No doubt the slang was spoken before it was written, but the point stands: 'sex' has had a long rapport with classification and a short one with screwing.

('Screw': first in print during the early eighteenth century. Suffolk County Court records, 1719: 'Mr. Boyd screwed Mr. Longs Maid of Charlestown.')

A far better word for intercourse itself is 'fuck'. Perhaps an ancient Germanic borrowing with older Indo-European origins, we find it in a sixteenth century Scottish courtier's poem. In William Dunbar's 1513 'A Man of Valour to his Fair Lady', a coiffed but clumsy youth shows he wants to sleep with his girlfriend: 'be his feirris he wald haue fukkit', or 'by his behaviour, he would have fucked'. The word turns up again in an Italian-English dictionary, under the definition of *fottere*: 'to iape, to sard, to fucke, to swive, to occupy'. In 1598 the English had some marvellous words for sex — but only 'fuck' is still with us.

No doubt this is partly the word's force: the breathy 'f' then percussive 'ck'. It is fun to say, and to pair with other words. (From my own Australia: 'fuckwit'.)

Put simply, as descriptions for copulation, I prefer the slang to the formal terminology. Of course, sex is more than fucking — this is the very basis of my philosophy. But insofar as I write about intercourse, I often choose the vulgar over the Vulgate.

This is partly an aesthetic decision. Most superficially, 'sex' is a clumsy word. It lacks the power of 'fuck', or even the levity of 'bonk' or 'roger'. (Humour is vital in the bedroom.) Even 'doing it' is better, with its suggestion of anonymous, private labours.

'Sex' also has a medical atmosphere to it; a mood of rubber gloves and forceps. (No judgement, if this is your fetish.) To say 'sex' rather than 'fuck' is often to prefer the physician's perspective to the lover's. This view is not false, but it is partial. It leaves out the first-person intimacy of screwing; the immediate feeling of self and other that arises here, amongst things — rather than from the Archimedean point noted by Nussbaum. This might seem aesthetic too, but it actually concerns a vision of reality I quietly encourage.

In *Why the World Does Not Exist*, philosopher Markus Gabriel writes that 'we prematurely create world pictures and in the process forget ourselves'. I write 'fuck' instead of 'sex' because I am trying not to forget myself.

Clowns

On Horror and Laughter in the Bedroom

In the hotel room, these newlyweds were almost naked. She, in a blue dress — no underwear. He, in a tieless shirt — no pants. Having rubbed her thigh, he pressed his penis against her vagina. There was a green stain on the light brown canopy above her. She stroked his penis, then pulled it to her vulva. He ejaculated on her.

These are the facts; the straightforward physical happenings. They are unambiguous and unremarkable. From a distance, they mean very little.

If we look more closely, this simplicity ends. The husband did not merely orgasm over his wife. He 'emptied himself over her in gouts ... filling her navel, coating her belly, thighs ... in tepid, viscous fluid.' This was not merely a climax — it is described to suggest discomfort and disgust: an organ is purging itself of lukewarm gunk.

In *On Chesil Beach*, Ian McEwan highlights the carnality of sex; the visceral reality of bodies in and on bodies. But he does so without a hint of titillation or bawdiness. His prose is deliberately physiological, turning erogenous zones into disembodied, disturbing bits ('his penis … repeatedly jabbing and bumping into and around her urethra'). As in Sartre's novel *Nausea*, this use of body parts keeps the scenes from feeling familiar. Everything is awkward and strange; flesh seems ugly and clumsy.

So, these passages leave me neither horny nor romantic. I do not groan or sigh — I cringe. And this prompts the obvious question: what genre is this explicit sex scene? Not erotica. Certainly not romance. Instead, it seems to shift between comedy and psychological thriller or horror.

In the first, Edward squirts semen while making noises like a waiter in a film, dropping dishes. This is the world of early sixties middle-class English cuisine — 'a slice of melon decorated by a single glazed cherry'. In the second, Florence feels his cum cooling on her skin, wipes herself with a pillow, then flees to the beach. This is the world of early sixties English middle-class matrimony, in which husbands and wives are each alone in their anxious naivety.

What makes *On Chesil Beach* so powerful is its refusal to give up on either atmosphere. The story is genuinely funny *and* genuinely creepy — *and* genuinely tragic.

Slippery

My point is not simply that the novel moves between derisory and gross scenes; first a cumshot, then a heaving gorge. This certainly happens, but it is not what makes *On Chesil Beach* exemplary. Instead, the sex is both hilarious and abhorrent, and this is a more universal ambiguity.

Take Edward's orgasm. Ejaculating on lovers is typically taken as a kind of dominance: whether you salivate or retch, taking a man's cum is seen as submissive. But Edward did not mean to squirt all over Florence; he did not mean to orgasm *at all*. He put it off once by thinking about Prime Minister Harold MacMillan ('he was everything that was not sex'), but Florence touching his cock was too much. Edward failed.

As Simone de Beauvoir notes in *The Second Sex*, penises are as much proof of biological tyranny as they are of freedom. Yes, the man can grow hard, thrust, and orgasm at all the right moments. This is the ideal of virility (which need not be heterosexual at all). But he can also get a boner during dinner, come too quickly, or fail to become erect at all. He can also be profoundly ashamed of his lust — at least afterwards. 'Man glories in the phallus when he thinks of it as transcendence ... as a means for taking possession of the other,' de Beauvoir wrote, 'but he is ashamed of it when he sees it as merely passive flesh through which he is the plaything of the dark forces of life.' The very same organ, even doing the very same things, can be laudatory or mocking.

This hardly needs proving, but cocks can also be funny. Think of Aristophanes' play *Lysistrata*, in which the women of Greece avoid sex until the men agree to an armistice. In one scene, a Spartan herald is talking to an Athenian magistrate about their celibacy — both with enormous erections. 'And that's why you've come,' the judge asks of the Spartan, 'hiding a spear in your clothes?' (The actors wore huge leather knobs.) As the French essayist Michel de Montaigne noted almost twenty centuries after Aristophanes, the penis so often 'thrusts itself forward inopportunely', until we ask it to stand stiff.

Edward's semen, described as 'slime from another body', is similarly changeable. There is nothing necessarily gross about seminal fluid. Yes, it can be felt as oozing clammily, or tasted as sour; it can be felt as shaming or violating (from Marilyn French's feminist classic *The Women's Room*: 'the salty stinging semen burned her throat'). But plenty of lovers enjoy cum. In her memoirs, Catherine Millet praises oral over vaginal sex because the mouth is more sensitive to touch and flavour. 'In the final phase,' she writes, 'you taste the sperm' — and this, for her, is a good thing. Krissy Kneen's short story 'The Dream of the Fisherman's Wife' is dripping with ejaculate, including an Alsatian's, pony's and octopus's. Love and lust are a miracle of sorts, turning goop into celebratory wine.

Were Florence wet, her arousal could be equally ambiguous. For centuries, men have vilified the vagina; treated it as ugly and dirty. The medieval theologian John Bromyard famously described woman as 'a temple built over a sewer', perhaps aping the theologian Tertullian. Witness the misogynistic metaphors: filth and fluidity. De Beauvoir observed how many men, including doctors, saw the vagina as a wound, festering and weeping. Even French philosopher Georges Bataille, in other ways so progressive about sexuality, continued this conservative idea. Yet the very same brackish seep is (rightly) championed by many.

Jeanette Winterson in *Written on the Body*: 'she opens and shuts like a sea anemone. She's refilled each day with fresh tides of longing.' What is vulgar to the pious patriarch is sexy to the horny lover.

Elsewhere, cum and juices are the stuff of everything from guffaws to wry smiles. In author Linda Jaivin's short story 'The Road to Gundagai', a lecturer in women's studies finds her car broken down by the Big Merino: a giant concrete sheep, just off a highway. Eventually, a trucker arrives to help. She has never fucked a man with less than a Master's degree, yet she is 'absolutely wetting [her] pants' at this tanned, reeking lunk. The mood is erotic, yes. But also comedic: her lubrication is at odds with her theory.

In short: the meaning of sexual parts and stuff is slippery. The most obvious bulge or wet patch can be horny in the hotel room, offensive in the office cubicle, and chucklesome in the courtroom. To say that McEwan's fictional fucking is ambiguous is simply to say that it is realistic (if not simple realism).

Moods

Life is always ambiguous in this way, shifting as we shift. As Martin Heidegger argued in *Being and Time*, a different state of mind appears as a different world. This is not because we somehow drape our feelings over things, like a canopy erected over a bed. For Heidegger, things always appear to us in light of our disposition. We exist in a thoroughly humanised cosmos. The German philosopher called the mood, or *Stimmung*, 'disclosive': it offers the universe to us in such and such a way, or not at all. 'Having a mood,' he wrote, 'brings Being to its "there".' In other words, the reality of any situation is thoroughly suffused with significance. In this way, we never meet things (or ourselves) outside of our own temper — even an aloof atmosphere is still an atmosphere, which highlights some things, while dimming others.

This is why even slight stimuli prompt enormous changes. Think of smells and sounds. D once kissed me on her parents' porch, pushing me against the warm red-brick wall. Many years later, strawberry chapstick brings this back, along with that whole adolescent milieu of fumbling and bumbling; along with the fine blonde down on her breasts, and the urgency of her tongue. The same smell on a taxi driver? No such Proustian journeys in that state of mind. In Krissy Kneen's short story 'Susanna', the eponymous hero is hiding in her neighbour's closet, watching him fuck an escort. Susannah masturbates avidly as she watches. But when the prostitute's 'heightened shrieks' seem fake, Susannah's arousal is 'suddenly deflated like a balloon'. She wants it all to stop, and her only urge is to use the bathroom. The mood is gone.

Think also of this line from Carmen Maria Machado's unsettling short story 'Inventory': 'We got high and fucked and I accidentally fell asleep with my hand inside of her.' The fisting evokes lust; the enjoyment of filling and being filled. And this is no doubt heightened by the drugs. But the lingering image is one of pleasant exhaustion and the quiet intimacy of sleep. The same two women in the same bed, on the same night: but the mood turns radically. (In fact, the whole tale involves a haunting shift of atmosphere.)

Which brings us back to Chesil beach. The state of mind is what changes for Florence when she is covered in cum. Her cautiously adventurous and briefly aroused love turns immediately to horror: the slime is too much. She wants to flee, because her whole universe suddenly drips with malice. Similarly, the state of mind is what changes for Edward when Florence leaves him. Instead of being a nervous but tender seducer, he becomes the jilted loner; the failure, surrounded by nothing but rejection and mockery. And these moods are invisible to one another: she can only see his macho posturing, and he her contemptuous coldness. Each is imprisoned within their transformed mood. The *Stimmung* is their sudden anger after weeks of cheer, and his sullen silence as she walks away. And then they are done, forever.

Unexpected Copulation

What are these moods about? And why are they so strong? Sex can be especially horrific or funny because of its paradoxes.

The magistrate with a boner, the feminist scholar wet over a trucker, the fantasy Prime Minister easing an erection — these are all examples of strife between notions. Putting it this way seems odd, as humour is often taken to be purely emotional. But it cannot work without some logic. To get a joke, we must understand what we are looking at — and also understand why it does not quite work. More specifically, much humour relies on some kind of mismatch, muddle, or contradiction. Philosopher Michael Clark put it stiffly in an essay for *Philosophy*, 'if an event/state of affairs etc. amuses someone, then he sees it as involving the incongruous subsumption of one or more instances under a single concept.' Samuel Johnson made the same point in *The Rambler* magazine, but made it funny: 'wit, you know, is the unexpected copulation of ideas'.

Not every incongruity will be laughable, and even the funny incongruities will not be funny for everyone. But part of all laughter is some discord between ideas. Even if the ideas are unspoken and unconscious, they are there: making sense (or not) of the world and ourselves.

Take Edward's premature ejaculation. Here, his own vision of himself clashes with reality. Instead of being the conquering stud, using his cock masterfully to delight his wife, he is a lump of spasming meat. This is funny because of the enormous distance between the two ideas; between Edward as glorious monarch of Florence's maidenhead, and Edward as a squirting fool. This is perhaps what French philosopher Henri Bergson, in his *Laughter*, called the 'mechanical encrusted on the living'. While Bergson saw this as the font of all comedy, it is better understood as one kind of incongruity: between concepts of freedom and necessity, spirit and flesh.

Edward's cum is also incongruous, because it is slimy. Putting aside Sartre's bizarre gender musings in *Being and Nothingness* — slime is 'feminine revenge', you see — he was right that this substance is odd. Neither a liquid nor a solid, it seems to slip away from our day-to-day physical notions. Like vomit, shit and blood, slime also is something inside that we meet outside; something invisible made visible; something that is very much mine but also quickly alien to me. Because of this, anything that sprays, oozes, drips from us can be a hoot.

And yet: pulsing organs and slime can also be shocking. Not because sex is sinful or evil, but because incongruity is also the stuff of horror. In fiction and life, these contradictions can be gross, eerie, terrifying. Take that epitome of suave, seductive power, the vampire. Dead but living, human yet animalistic, civilised and bloodsucking — Dracula is a paradox. This makes him sexy, as the uncanny has undoubtable charisma. But it also makes him unsettling: a prompt for crawling skin and clenching guts. Likewise for werewolves, zombies, cyborgs. These monsters, like much in horror, are all conceptually jumbled — what philosopher Noël Carroll calls 'impure': interstitial, incomplete, incompatible.

Because they overturn our everyday categories, they prompt a flinch or shiver.

What shifts us from laughter to fear? Threat. The very same monsters that have us shuddering when dangerous are hilarious when benign. This applies to fanged beasts, lumbering automatons, empty ghouls, but also to penises, vaginas, and their fluids.

Florence flees from Edward's semen, not simply because it is slimy, but because she feels bullied by him; because his masculine desire calls to mind her father's — and so his abuse. Witness McEwan's language: 'its alien milkiness ... dragged with it the stench of a shameful secret'. This is comedy quickly becoming horror.

In other words, the very thing that makes sex an invitation to philosophy — what I described earlier as 'plaited and puzzling' existence — is also what makes it a muddle of genres. Our moods shift so quickly, and change us so profoundly, because lust involves strong but strange ideas. The world of desire is not necessarily perverse, but certainly extraordinary.

The Backwards Step

The laugh and the cringe are both responses to the paradoxes of sex, its organs and fluids. But they are not *equal* responses.

Perhaps because they suggest genres — comedy, horror, psychological thriller, and so on — chortling and alarm seem equivalent. They just look like the varied emotions of a varied library. And it is true that neither response is ethically or technically superior. Both Sophocles and Aristophanes dramatised sexual incongruity — neither was more edifying or masterful than the other.

But for audiences and lovers, laughter is special — at least when we laugh at ourselves. To weep, flinch, or rage is to be committed to the world. Whether the world is fictional or not, we respond to it with seriousness. Florence's gorge fills with bile as the cum cools on her; Edward's blood pressure rises as his wife leaves him and his flaccid cock in the hotel room — and we feel along with them, if not as them. We are, as they are, *there*: stuck in a universe that disgusts or discomfits us. It all *matters*, and this cannot be undone or unthought.

When we laugh, it matters less — if not absolutely, then in that moment. In laughter, another incongruity occurs: between the overwhelming to-and-fro of existence, and an aloof observation of this existence. There are familiar metaphors to describe this: heaviness and lightness, lowliness and flight, proximity and distance. In 'The Absurd', philosopher Thomas Nagel speaks simply of life, and a 'backwards step'. Whatever trope we use to make sense of this laughter, it makes sense because it is a fundamental part of our psyche. We are creatures who can become aware of our creatureliness; who can recognise how mired we are, from within this mire — and find it hilarious. Nietzsche put it this way in *The Gay Science*: 'precisely because we are at bottom grave and serious human beings — really more weights than human beings — nothing does us as much good as a fool's cap'. Strange splits in the world — slime, dignified folly, sweet violation, enjoyable agony, and so on — invite strange splits in us, and we can deal with these cuts by laughing.

This humour is vital. Instead of feeling burdened by existence, we gain a buoyancy. Yes, these are the same hackneyed metaphors, but the state of mind they highlight is real and good: it keeps us from breaking under the gravity of fear, grief, regret — or from doing something horrible to ease this density.

In my fantasy version of *On Chesil Beach*, Florence is still shocked, but Edward is able to shrug off his macho millstone. As he comforts his wife, he chuckles supportively: not at her nausea, but at his own failings. He is strong enough to snort at his own weakness: now, and in the coming years. This saves him from the rage that lets Florence walk away from their relationship; saves his wife from her violated shame. His laugh says: *we are not alone here, you and I, in this absurd world.* Perhaps their marriage continues, and — despite the suffering that must always be — they are well. They smile often, and teach their children this very moral art.

We need to laugh at ourselves because — at some point, however distant — we are all Edward and Florence. Or Edward and Edward, or Florence and Florence, or some tangle of each or neither (not everyone is a 'he' or 'she'). Even with eager consent, sex can be awkward or anxious, over too soon or dragging on. It can be the wrong kind of fucking, or the right kind with the wrong lover. Even having screwed well, I might find myself like Schopenhauer's stereotypical man: 'after all his lofty, heroic, and endless attempts to further his own pleasure he has obtained but little'. Meanwhile, youth can make us premature, and age flaccid or dry; poor health can leave us aching for it — or just aching.

And then there are uppers and downers, pills and drams. Some believe variety keeps sex interesting — alas, there are a variety of ways to fail.

This is why wit is needful: to keep enjoying sex, despite reality.

Moods Do Not Believe in Each Other

Of course, to laugh in this way we have to feel safe; to not feel distraught like Florence or demeaned like Edward. Or, rather: we have to be *able* to feel otherwise. Once we have quivered or cringed, how might we wear the fool's cap?

Importantly, this is not a question of smarts. Yes, our sense of humour matures with our minds. Babies giggling at peek-a-boo are learning about unexpected events; toddlers waving their genitals in kindergarten are making unexpected events happen. (Confession: I was the toddler.) Incongruity requires cognitive development to understand. But for adults confronting the absurdities of sex, levity is conceptually simple — the complications are typically emotional. Put another way: this is not about getting the joke, this is about finding it funny.

I am also not interested in mockery or schadenfreude here — laughing at, rather than with. Of course we can snort at others' expense, especially those we dislike or distrust. We enjoy both their loss of dignity and our own safety from it. Philosophers like Thomas Hobbes believed that all comedy came from this: the so-called 'superiority' theory. In *Leviathan*, he wrote that sniggerers find 'some deformed thing in another, by comparison whereof they suddenly applaud themselves.' But Hobbes was wrong, his idea of humour as one-sidedly pessimistic as his idea of humanity itself. The English philosopher missed not only puns and nonsense, but also laughing at ourselves. We do this, not because we are superior, but because we recognise that we are all 'deformed things'.

So, the clown here is myself — and I want to laugh. But between me and comedy is my own state of mind: wrath, shame, odium, paralysis, or some other enemy of lust. As American philosopher Ralph Waldo Emerson noted, these atmospheres are so often mutually exclusive. Not simply because we feel differently in each, but because our whole outlook is different. 'Moods,' he wrote in his essay 'Circles', 'do not believe in each other.' If I am hostile from awkward celibacy or numbed by failed late-night fumbling, carnal joy does not exist. Emerson's phrase sums up Edward's fall from erect elation to flaccid anger: 'I am God in nature; I am a weed by the wall.' I can always think of joyous sex, of course; can bring to mind ideas of gentle intimacy or avid boning. But these ideas will be abstract, with none of the *Stimmung*'s disclosive power. And without this power, thinking of humour is no humour at all.

In this light, the quest of the miserable lover is to somehow change their world; to do away with fact for what seems, at that moment, like fiction.

Third Natures

Alas, there is no user's manual for moods; no quick fix to move from melancholy to joviality. In a letter to a friend, the art critic John Ruskin once remarked that 'One can't be angry when one looks at a Penguin.' Ruskin was no stranger to sexual shame, and perhaps needed a marital pick-me-up long before his very public divorce. But who will store, along with the vibrator and lubricant, a flightless bird?

There is no easy rule here; no law that tells us how to be funny, or even when to. Even without malice, we can harm with levity. In Milan Kundera's *The Unbearable Lightness of Being*, the womaniser Tomas is caught cheating on his girlfriend, Tereza. For months, his head has stunk of another woman's groin. After all his sneaky shower scrubbing, he had forgotten the lover who asked him to fuck her with the crown of his head. 'All he could do was laugh a silly laugh,' Kundera writes, 'and head for the bathroom to wash his hair.' This is so absurd that Tomas chortles. But none of this is actually funny — not in the fiction as written, or in life as lived. Though Kundera does not say, I expect Tereza is hurt by her beloved's laughter. The man who lies to her is now chuckling at his own failure to be canny. His guilt remains, and it is hurtful.

Sometimes levity comes with danger. Witness the countless jokes or skits portraying a woman who is actually a man: the 'ladyboy' shocking some straight dude with her cock, the extravagant queen with the prominent moustache. And this is not just a modern, European trope. In seventeenth-century China, provincial tutor Pu Songling portrayed the same shock for laughs. In his tale 'The Male Concubine', Songling tells us a rich man from Yangzhou bought a pretty teenager. But when he began to grope her, he found 'to his shock and horror ... "she" was in fact a boy.' This is often played for giggles in literature, cinema and on television, but it is also used to frighten: think of Gotham's Joker, with his mincing manner and 'sissy' voice. Our two gender categories are so seemingly natural, that anyone who transgresses is either a clown or a monster — that is, either hilarious or horrifying.

They ought not to be so. Throughout history, there have been other categories. India's famous *Kama Sutra* casually speaks of a 'person of a third nature', neither man nor woman. Within the animistic Bugis culture of Sulawesi, the *bissu* were (and are) born intersex or with ambiguous physiology, and took up female customs. Importantly, the *bissu* were not seen as lowly or vile. They were religious authorities, who had the ears of kings and divinities. 'As the *bissu* bring together woman and man in one person,' writes Asian studies scholar Sharyn Graham Davies, 'they can mediate between humans and gods through blessings.' Alongside the *bissu*, the Bugis world recognised another four genders: men, women, female men, and male women. Given their transcendence, the *bissu* were still paradoxical: it was *because* they combined basic concepts that they were elevated beyond everyday life. But this did not lead to hilarity or nausea, because it was granted a new concept: the guide, the shaman, the priest.

Similar pluralism existed across the world. This was not only in south-east Asia and the subcontinent — where the *Hijra* of India still live — but also in Africa, Polynesia, and the Americas. The Maya, for example, had 'men-women' and 'women-men', and art historian Matthew Looper argues that kings often performed as third gender maize and moon deities. Their temple architecture also mirrored this triadic logic, with third spaces for ambiguous genders. These discoveries led archaeologist Miranda Stockett, in an essay for *World Archaeology*, to conclude that our modern binary concepts are just too simplistic to do justice to ancient Mesoamerica.

Importantly, they are also too simplistic for today. As philosopher Robin Dembroff argues, the usual dualism is not only untrue for many people, but also unjust. It fails to make sense of the extraordinary miscellany of gender performances, and it treats full human beings as merely freaks. It turns everything from brief transvestism to life-long transexuality into fakery; it makes their whole being a kind of swindle or devilry. This stigma is painful, alienating, and often precedes violence. Our taken-for-granted categories, Dembroff writes in *Aeon* magazine, 'make life into a tightrope where one misstep or just bad luck ends in unemployment, harassment, rape, beatings or even death.'

None of this shows that sexual physiology is incidental or inconsequential. There are still penises and vaginas, testes and ovaries, neurotransmitters and hormones. Far from being slavering beasts, men actually think more clearly with the right levels of testosterone. A review of the literature by Dr Jeremy Hua and colleagues reported improvements to older men's 'memory, attention, and executive function' with testosterone supplements. Women tend to be hornier after their periods — when they are most fertile. 'Coincidence?' writes anthropologist Robert Martin in *How We Do It*. 'I don't think so.' We are constantly nudged and shoved, often without our knowing, by our biology.

But part of our biology is extraordinary psychological and social openness: genes do not wholly determine who and what we are. The *bissu* and their like reveal that gender has no natural or god-given relationship with physical sex. Even for those whose bits and selves dovetail, the fit is rarely perfect — and often loose. 'In every human being a vacillation from one sex to the other takes place,' Virginia Woolf wrote in *Orlando*, 'and often it is only the clothes that keep the male or female likeness, while underneath the sex is the very opposite of what it is above.' There is no cosmic plan or law that states: dick means masculine, pussy means feminine. And these ideas themselves are troublesome. 'Masculine' and 'feminine' are traits that *all* of us can have, so why are they gendered at all? Some might quibble, saying that men *ought* to have only masculine traits, and women feminine. But we cannot pluck a cultural 'ought' from a biological 'is', and there is no deity passing us such a bauble. In short: our gender binary is a caricature of humanity, not a faithful portrait.

So, suppose I am seduced by a nonbinary lover. Perhaps I respond to their drollery, and knowledge of the Batman mythos, and burgundy lipstick, and teal coat. And perhaps I kiss off that lipstick and pull off that coat and — suddenly their ambiguity is not ambiguous at all. If I cringe or laugh at them, and forget their wit and cute nerdisms, I am wrong: ontologically, but also morally.

Ontology concerns what is: our most basic ideas of existence. Typically, these seem so ordinary that they cannot be questioned — until they are. Think of 'atom', which comes from the Greek, and means something that cannot be split. One of the twentieth century's great ontological revolutions was literally dividing this indivisible thing. What seemed like an eternal verity turned out to be an abstraction. Reality was famously more weird. And the same is true of 'man' and 'woman'. These seemingly fundamental categories are rightly blown to pieces by nonbinary people. Their mere existence is an explosion, which is why I might mistakenly flinch or cackle — I cannot cope with what they destroy.

I am morally wrong here, because I turn their existence into pure Hobbesian comedy or horror. Morality is no simple thing, but at the very least it requires recognition: seeing another human being *as* another human being. I have to overcome my own selfish urges and fantasies, and try to witness another's psychological nuance and social complexity. By treating my stylish Batman connoisseur as a clown — to be feared or mocked — I give up on this ethical project.

The joke is on me. How foolish am I, expecting reality to mimic my binary fantasies?

Eutrapelia

So, it is not only moods that shift — it is ethical circumstances. Even if we are not Hobbesians, laughter can alienate and abuse as much as it welcomes and protects. We have to be careful with our jibes.

Because of this, there is an art to comedy; to finding the right levity in the right moment, in the right situation. This is what the Greeks called *eutrapelia*, which philosopher WD Ross translates as 'ready-wittedness'. Literally, it meant turning well, or easily — a kind of mental agility or suppleness.

It was first praised by the Athenian statesman Pericles in his famous funeral oration, left to us by the historian Thucydides. The Athenians were neither dogmatic nor flippant, said the orator. They were independent citizens, and each one achieved this with 'exceptional grace and exceptional versatility' (*eutrapelos*). True or false, the portrait Pericles left is an attractive one: an 'easy mind', which avoids both dogmatism and caprice.

Some ninety years later, Aristotle praised *eutrapelia* in his *Nicomachean Ethics*. For Aristotle, morality was more than political or military duty. He sought a good life, which included leisure. As the Athenians spoke at parties or in the marketplace, they needed wit: the gift of tasteful and well-timed humour. As always, Aristotle put his morality neatly into three parts: an excess and deficiency to each side, with virtue in the middle. The ready-witted, in this, are neither buffoons nor boors. The first are always 'striving after humour at all costs' — this is the excess. The second 'neither make a joke themselves nor put up with those who do' — this is the deficiency. So, someone who has cultivated *eutrapelia* finds the mean between these extremes. They avoid being pedantic or otherwise dull, but do not become clowns in doing so. They have quips and puns, but not cruel jests or vulgar jibes.

Aristotle was a conservative, and his 'good and well-bred man' might not joke about fucking (let alone call it 'fucking'). But the gist is right, and works for the bedroom as much as for the symposium or *agora*: making light of things is a talent. This talent helps us to enjoy life, including our sex life. If we cannot find pleasure in the deed, we can gain some in laughter. And this can help, in turn, with the deed. Much is made of sexual acrobatics; of bent legs, arched backs, stretched arms. The 'lissom youth' is an ancient cliché. But we also need this litheness in our minds: to move from arousal, to shock or anger, to levity, and perhaps back to arousal — and to know when we cannot or should not.

And we need this virtue throughout our lives, not simply in adolescence or young adulthood. Because of the high stakes, *On Chesil Beach* makes much of the fated wedding night. And understandably: McEwan rightly labours to leave Florence and Edward ignorant of themselves and one another; to keep them alone, virginal and terrified. Even if this is more fable than historical truth, it is fair to the spirit of the age. But their hotel room muddles are not the only kind.

In his poem 'Elderly Sex', the American novelist John Updike compares screwing to a treasure hunt or circus act. Where once there were countless precious stones spilling out, now there might be one pearl — *might*. All of that effort, for so little? And so much care and concentration, stopped by a cold breeze or cleared throat? This is classic incongruity, and Updike allows us to smile if not laugh.

Likewise, in Ellen Bass's poem 'The Morning After' a middle-aged spouse stands at the bench, watching her partner making coffee. And making lunch. And making a call to their mother. But the night before, they were fucking. And this libidinous mood lingers with the narrator, along with the idea that sex gathers them together somehow — as a couple, and as individual selves. She wants that creaturely violence again, 'that brawl,/ that raw and radiant free-for-all.' But her bed-mate has gone — as if they were wearing a wig; were incognito in the kitchen. This is Alain Badiou's theory of love, exemplified: 'a construction, a life that is being made, no longer from the perspective of One but from the perspective of Two'. In this two, the narrator knows her beloved is back into their workaday checklists; that she is alone in her throbs and pulses; and that their lives together will continue nonetheless. It is a tender poem, thick with the adoration of decades. But it is also quietly funny, because of its instantly recognisable strife: between two moods, each of which is absolutely sovereign in that moment.

The point is not that older sex *must* be this way, but that newlyweds have no monopoly on lived paradox. We need *eutrapelia* because, for human beings, even leisure can be conflicted and contradictory — that is to say, can be laughable.

Aristotle offered no quick tips for developing ready-wittedness, and I have none myself. Yes, comedy is a craft, and tact is a virtue (so I am told) — and each can be learned, if not taught. And like all excellences, *eutrapelia* begins with what Aristotle called a 'kinship to virtue': a basic taste for goodness, encouraged early in life. Once we have this, though, wit must still be developed with practical wisdom; must be coaxed in various moods, with various intimates; must be discovered again in each generation, as mores change.

If *On Chesil Beach* suggests any general maxim, it is this: there is no escape from paradox. To have sex is to accept the possibility of ambiguity and ambivalence. This possibility need not be realised, of course. We can flee into mechanistic ideas of existence, or simplistic gender tropes; we can speak of 'easy quickies' and 'sluts who put out', and think no more. We can just be lucky for a while: good health, generous schooling, progressive crowds, and lovers whose kinks and libidos fit with ours. But eventually, in a moment of weakness or vulnerability, incongruity will find us. And when it does, we clowns ought to be prepared to laugh.

Bubbles

On the Fragility of Horniness

K held the whisk firmly, but only between her thumb and forefinger. It seemed loose this way; seemed more casual than her creased brow suggested. She wrote similarly: so seriously at every stiff joint, except where pen met skin. Hunched like this at the bench or kitchen table, she reminded me of Jan Steen's *Girl Eating Oysters*.

(K did not like oysters.)

Smiling briefly — more a tic than a grin — K turned yolk and glair to yellow froth. Then poured it smooth, added feta and dill. And we had an omelette.

We spoke about eggs and their need for pairings, and the discussion added to the flavour: common concentration worked like salt.

Afterwards, we walked to the bedroom, stopping to drop our jeans and such. It was warm. Spring or autumn warmth, in which the heat was merely a backdrop behind foreground living; not yet a monstrous thing in itself, burning skin and eucalypts.

During that afternoon, K held me between her thumb and forefinger. Loosely. Like a Dutch burgher holding an oyster to salt it.

After a few minutes, she paused.

And by 'paused', I mean K stopped and stared at me for perhaps twenty seconds. I mean little more than a moment. I mean far less time than it took her to turn eggs into omelette. But I also mean more than enough time for me to turn from luxuriating to shaking to gritting my teeth.

Frenulum

And then K

In anatomy, a frenulum is a fold of tissue. This seems trivial, but it is actually a glorious miniature.

finally

The diminutive of the Latin *frenum*, or 'bridle', a frenulum connects or restricts body parts. There is one under the tongue, which prevents the muscle from flexing too far. This can also become ulcerated after cunnilingus. There is another where the labia minora meet below the vagina.

and very deliberately

The penile frenulum is where the foreskin joins the head, or *glans* ('acorn'). While the foreskin is typically loose to allow movement back and forth, the frenulum is especially tight. In his 1838 *Manual of Descriptive and Pathological Anatomy*, German anatomist Johann Friedrich Meckel the Younger described the *frenulum glandis* as 'tense, short, and intimately united with the corresponding portion of the glans'.

though with no

In the womb, this intimate unity develops during the second trimester: the *glans* grows first, then the prepuce emerges to cover it. This takes approximately five weeks, and is typically completed by five months into the pregnancy — 'a fast process,' according to urology professor Luciano Favorito and colleagues.

exaggerated

For many babies, it takes little to undo these weeks: about five to ten minutes for circumcision. Here, the foreskin is often seen as superfluous; as a vestigial sack or curtain, which can be cut away for religious or aesthetic reasons without loss. But the prepuce is quite specialised, involving specific nerve types. New Zealand anatomist Ken McGrath compares the *glans* to the eye's cornea, and the foreskin to fingertips. Both are very responsive, but the former is clumsily so, while the latter enjoys careful discrimination. In his paper 'The Frenular Delta', McGrath observes that the frenulum is dense with Meissner's corpuscles, which 'mediate low-threshold and fine-touch sensation'. Put simply: the little bridle is more touchy than the acorn.

cinematic movements

Because of this, the frenulum can be essential for arousal and orgasm. In his pioneering 1847 textbook of applied anatomy, Austrian doctor and skull-collector Joseph Hyrtl observed that friction upon the frenulum led to 'the culminating point of the feeling of delight'. Hyrtl was a vitalist, who believed in a living force beyond mere physical stuff. He criticised contemporary materialists for reducing human experience to human physiology. 'How can the uniform gray matter,' he asked rhetorically in his rectoral address, 'give rise to such a diversity of mental life?' Nonetheless, even Hyrtl recognised that those few folds of skin and mucous membrane provided men with heightened gratification.

kissed

There are various ways to pleasure someone, obviously. We are not simply brains connected to a few oozing tumescences. But, for men, the little bridle is especially sensitive to touch. It offers, not simply pleasure, but a subtle continuum of bliss: a way to carefully offer or withhold stimulation. It can be used to slow or speed up rhythms; to shift attention from a diffuse erotic mood to a concentrated genital arousal; to take someone from plateau, to orgasm, to plateau.

my

In other words: the frenulum is a point of sexual control. It offers some mastery over another's state of mind.

frenulum.

On Teasing

In short: I was being teased. What did this feel like?

Falsely translated into prose, my psyche was saying something like: *this is not happening, this is still not happening, why is this not happening, perhaps this will never happen*. Note the 'this', which was foremost in my mind. To say that my consciousness — centred chiefly in my groin — was formed from lack suggests a void or cipher. But my mind was actually full: with K, her lips and tongue. So, by withdrawing herself, K made herself even more present to me. Witness Roland Barthes' description of loving, from *The Lover's Discourse*: 'you have gone (which I lament), you are here (since I am addressing you)'. Put another way, and with as little smug paradox as possible: I felt this absence as a very particular presence.

This, in turn, left me jittery, antsy, fidgety. In what ought to have been a languorous afternoon, I was neither calm nor straightforwardly aroused; neither settling into my own torpor, nor cheerily responsive to touch. Instead, I was overly aware of myself and K: stuck with uncomfortable unpredictability. I knew K's lips were gone (past), I hoped for them to return (future), and there was no way to unite these ideas. Barthes again: 'I know what the present, that difficult tense, is: a pure portion of anxiety.'

Here, I am not endorsing that foolish trope of femininity: the prick-tease. Many of women's supposed tricks are the fantasies of entitled men; of those for whom the world is supposed to move immediately from wish to fulfilment.

Teasing transcends the gender of the teased or teasing. It is a feeling common to anyone capable of lust and its frustrations. Yes, at that moment I felt like Cinesias from Aristophanes' *Lysistrata*, on his cock: 'Poor little lad ... he pines and peeks./ Our lovely girl has proved a curse .../ A nurse to cherish him, a nurse!' Yet I also sympathised with the maid in Carol Ann Duffy's poem 'Warming Her Pearls', who wears her employer's necklace to warm it. After all her intimacies with this lady, the maid goes to her attic bed alone: the pearls become cold, but she does not. This is not a pause during fucking, but the logic is similar: the pain of the just-out-of-reach.

And yet, for all these complaints, I very much wanted to keep reaching; wanted K *not* to kiss me. I wanted the ache to continue, because it was enjoyable. Or, rather: the absence of pleasure was its own kind of pleasure. This is intimated by the etymology of 'tease' itself, which comes from Old English. To *taes* was 'to separate or pull asunder the fibres of,' the *Oxford English Dictionary* reports, 'to comb or card (wool, flax, etc.) in preparation for spinning'. The metaphor is interesting: teasing suggests scraping or rasping, but for some worthwhile end. Irritation with goodwill.

So, if I was the wool or flax, what was being made of me? Not some stronger fabric. Certainly nothing more fine or fancy. I was more like a string played by a maestro. More like Vulcan's bronze wires, which trapped Mars and Venus while they screwed — though I was the couple *and* the chains (Ovid: 'he made them so that they would yield to the slightest touch, and to the smallest movement').

In short: by teasing me, K left me with a more quickened existence. Yes, I was anxious — but it was *my* anxiety; an anxiety that left me taut and reverberating.

Scheherazade

So, my creaturely sensitivity had a wisdom to it: of presence and absence; of accepting just enough for wish, but not enough for fulfilment. This is the structure of teasing.

Yet there was a larger structure to that afternoon, which transcended physiology and its throbs. Witness the omelette before, and then coffee after; witness the intimacy before that allowed for K's nous and my expectation of it. That single kiss was oriented to climax in the short term, but togetherness in the longer term.

Put another way: this blowjob was a brief story within stories. And this pattern is ubiquitous in life and fiction.

This is not simply because we are entertained by tales, but because they make sense of our lives — and how we live them.

In the early twentieth century, the German philosopher Edmund Husserl argued that we do not simply live in time, but actually *make* time. Temporality is part of our psychology. We pull along our pasts behind in the present, while seeking the future. We are continually sorting ideas into 'now' and 'then', based not on abstract clock times, but on how we think and feel about these ideas. This does not mean we introduce some foreign logic to time — this is *our* time. 'It is no more alien to time than the curving banks are alien to the river, or the potter's hands to the clay,' philosopher David Carr writes in *Time, Narrative, and History*. 'Mere sequence … is not something we could ever experience.'

In this way, consciousness has a narrative character. This is what literary scholar David Herman and linguist Becky Childs call, in the journal *Style*, 'a pattern-forming cognitive system that organizes all sequentially experienced structure'. Beginnings, middles, ends; origins, journeys, destinations; seductions, lovemaking, climaxes — these are how we knead the world into consumable lumps. These might be deceptively firm or clean; might neglect all kinds of ambiguity or transience. (As I argue in *The Art of Reading*, we ought to sometimes suppress our own greedy appetite for stories.) Still, they are fundamental to our humanity.

And these narratives, in turn, always take place within and alongside others. As philosopher Alasdair MacIntyre observes in *After Virtue*, we cannot make sense of one another without stories: not only of seconds or minutes, but also of years, centuries, millennia. In this way, what

seems like a kind of authorial egotism actually asks for
humility. We come into a world of tales, yes. But many are
ancient, and most are lived and told by strangers. 'In my
drama ... I am Hamlet or Iago or at least the swineherd
who may yet become a prince,' MacIntyre writes, 'but to
you I am only A Gentleman or at best Second Murderer,
while you are my Polonius or my Gravedigger'.

Because these stories are so primal, they too can
cause anxiety. In fact, they require anxiety to work. This
is not simply in horror tales or thrillers — all narratives
involve some discomfort or disquieting tension. Consider
Alessandro Baricco's *Silk*. I might simply describe the novel
thus: a French merchant never screws the Japanese woman
he fetishises. This summary offers a true description,
but it is not a storied description; it does not make us
wait, as the tale moves from premise to conclusion. It
is only because I have read of Hervé's years of yearning
that the denouement moves me ('drawn on the water, he
seemed to see the inexplicable spectacle, light, that had
been his life'). It is only because I have longed to learn
of Hervé — phrase by phrase, paragraph by paragraph
— that his longing exists for me. I give myself freely to
this frustration, because it offers the greater pleasure of
striving and achieving.

This is why *One Thousand and One Nights* is such a
sexy collection. Yes, it begins with fucking, and continues
this way for hundreds of pages ('he withdrew from her
and after a restorative pause, he returned fifteen times').
But it is also sexy because its basic premise is teasing:
stories, within stories, within stories, until I forget what
led to which.

Scheherazade keeps King Shahriyar anxious about her
tales, and in so doing keeps herself and her sister alive

— and me entertained. Michael Austin, writing in the journal *Philosophy and Literature*:

> To be human is to tell stories, to experience
> pleasure in their construction, and to feel anxiety
> at their interruption; and, like Scheherazade, we
> will cease to exist as a species the moment that
> we have no more stories to tell.

In this light, K holding and kissing me was a bodily narrative; a (gripping) story, in which the telling was physical rather than verbal. Yet in teasing me, she was doing what all good storytellers have done: making her audience wait.

The Membrane

But not wait too much.

Suppose K took another thirty seconds; then, clearing her throat, observed that the low-fat feta was not briny or tangy enough; then began itemising a shopping list. These were certainly part of our common personal narratives: did they belong in the bedroom?

Confronted with these quotidian facts, I would have lost the plot, quite literally. The narrative would have ended early. Not because it was false, but because it was no longer gripping; because my anxiety was suddenly about the storytelling, not the story itself.

In the language of American sociologist Erving Goffman, I would no longer be 'engrossed'. In his lecture 'Fun in Games', Goffman discussed the very particular dynamics of these formal, face-to-face gatherings

— what he called 'encounters'. They involve common concentration; some focal point, to which everyone is oriented. This focal point is highly symbolic, giving words and gestures extra meaning. Participants are aware of one another's faces, and sensitive to communication. As these suggest, encounters have a 'we' logic to them; a sense that we are not alone, but part of a shared world. And these worlds are secondary, not primary — new universes which occur amidst the workaday one. These encounters often begin and end with recognisable customs, prompting a shift in our consciousness.

Here, Goffman was describing football, duelling, and soirees — but also fucking. He recognised that playing games and lovemaking were not exactly the same, observing in a footnote that 'substitutes cannot ordinarily be brought in' during the latter. Still, they were close enough to be enlightening. Screwing well — like scoring a goal or first blood, or hosting a clever party — means exercising my talents in a somewhat fickle universe. These talents might be thrusting and parrying, or they might simply be breathing and concentrating. The important thing is that we strive, and by striving give ourselves to a common narrative. If the outcome is absolutely determined, I get bored. If the outcome is random, my skills are useless. A good encounter will essentially tell a story with some doubt, and give everyone involved a chance to play hero within this ambiguity.

When this happens, Goffman said, the encounter forms a kind of 'membrane' between itself and ordinary life. It keeps the primary world at a distance. But as the biological metaphor suggests, this is not done entirely, or once and for all. Instead, a successful encounter is a continual to-and-fro between primary and secondary worlds. Some things are excluded wholly: discussions of groceries during a blowjob, for example. (If this is your kink, my apologies — list those goods without shame, friend.) Some things are changed: light is lowered or filtered, perhaps; kisses slowed or quickened. And often the authority during the encounter — judge, referee, host, lover — will have to be spontaneous: deciding when to speak or be silent, when to laugh or be serious.

Suppose the doorbell had rung that afternoon — after the kiss, but before the cheese chat. This would have been the primary world entering suddenly into the secondary, what Goffman called an 'incident'. It might have prompted K to check the door hastily, perhaps look for a package or card in the letterbox. Everyday doubts and regrets might have ruined my buzz. Instead of euphoria, I would have felt dysphoria: 'self-conscious, overinvolved, and acutely uncomfortable.' In this way, the encounter would have simply ended; the secondary world would have dissolved into the primary.

For Goffman, such incidents ask for 'integration': the annoyance has to be 'redefined and its reconstituted meaning integrated'. Put simply: we have to change the incident to fit the encounter, or the encounter to fit the incident, or both. So, to integrate our doorbell, K might have joked with me ('get dressed, the postman knows about us') then continued, making the interruption part of the story's internal world. This would have maintained trust between us, and done away with the distraction. We would have been together in our laughter. There would have been tension, yes, but of the erotic sort: within the encounter, rather than between me and my focal points. Suspense, not estrangement.

Obviously, tension comes in various kinds — and we respond variously to it. During sex, serious generalised anxiety affects straight more than queer women. Also, our distractions can be gendered in content, if not in structure. When sexual problems arise, men are more likely to be thinking about clumsy or weak performance and poor erections, women about psychological alienation and abuse. Think of Japanese author Nagata Kabi's recent *manga* memoir *My Lesbian Experience with Loneliness*. A lonely virgin in her twenties, Kabi hires an escort to help her cultivate her adult intimacy — including her first kiss. The other woman is gentle and encouraging, but Kabi cannot get over her own discomfort and disassociation. Her worries quickly end her lust. 'What was I?' she thinks, as the escort licks her. 'Someone who failed at being a person?' For all its cultural and psychological idiosyncrasies, Kabi's story is representative.

Still, precariousness is our common lot. In a paper for the *Archives of Sexual Behaviour*, Pedro Nobre and José Pinto-Gouveia report 'a certain uniformity in men and women,' when it comes to psychological disruptions. For both traditional genders, the waylaying notions are automatic, and lead to thoughts of failure, then to feelings of sadness — which end the erotic atmosphere. No such research exists yet for transgender lovers, alas. But studies do consistently find that being profoundly ill-at-ease with one's body is correlated with chronic sadness and stress, both of which stifle desire or orgasm. They also find that hormone therapy and surgery lead to higher levels of sexual satisfaction. Urologist Jochen Hess and colleagues report that trans women's orgasms were more intense after surgery, perhaps because 'they were able to experience orgasm for the first time in a body that matched their perception'. In short: they were aroused without estrangement.

So, many encounters are flimsy, and barbed reality can easily 'poke through the thin sleeve of immediate reality,' as Goffman put it. Because of this, we are all alike in the fragility of our worlds; in the weakness of our membranes. Sexual stories are zealous and ubiquitous, but it is very simple to lose the plot.

This is even more so for teasing, which ramps up euphoria with anxiety — but also elevates the danger of dysphoria. The more sexual tension, the more likely the tension will become too much altogether. Even if we arrange everything just right — the omelette cooked, the linen fresh, the room warm — our psyches might not be up to it. The thrilling tale becomes a drudge or bore; from frenular jolts to just fed up.

Good sex is a bubble, teased out and kept carefully from popping.

Mrs Dalloway

I now move from explanation to celebration.

As encounters, our trysts are frail. And frailty does not always ask for gentleness. Sometimes, to avoid bursting the membrane we are threatening or forceful. At other times, we are coaxing or coddling. Either way, we have to be careful and deft. This involves concern for our lovers' needs and wants, and a sense of their mood. We cannot know exactly how they feel, but we can learn how to help them feel it. If not maestros, we can become adepts of sexual atmospheres.

In 'Fun in Games', Goffman describes excellent party hosts, who invite complementary guests, and know how to keep them lively and cheery. Well before a single glass of wine is poured, they make sure the guests are familiar enough to get along, but not boring to one another. 'So we find that the euphoria function for a sociable occasion,' Goffman wrote, 'resides somewhere between little social difference and much social difference.' And while the party runs, they too run from guest to guest, group to group. They highlight witticisms, banish ill-feelings. They have the 'charm, tact, or presence of mind' to turn awkward confessions into forgotten gaffes; to nudge the shy into conversation and push the bellicose into silence.

Such talents are widely enjoyed, but often trivialised. Why? Because they are gendered as feminine, and are therefore lesser. As political scientist Anne Phillips and historian Barbara Taylor observe in their paper 'Sex and Skill', even when men and women do the same kinds of jobs, their work is often divided into 'skilled' and 'unskilled' respectively. 'The work of women is often deemed inferior,' they write, 'because it is women who do it.' Just as women's factory labours have been scorned as simple, women's domestic roles have been judged as low drudgery or frippery; as not 'real' work, deserving of respect or even remuneration. They need to be done — but not to be lauded.

One of the joys of Virginia Woolf's novel *Mrs Dalloway* is its salute to Clarissa Dalloway. She is seen as a shallow society wife; as someone defined by whom she is married to, rather than by her own existence. And it is true that she has neither political nor employment experience; she is neither a statesman like her husband, nor a worker like her servants. But she does have her own vocation: parties. She brings guests together, and does so beautifully — like the tolling of Big Ben. 'She made her drawing-room a sort of meeting-place,' thinks Clarissa's old suitor Peter Walsh, 'she had a genius for it.' We all must confront death, like Woolf's poor Septimus Smith; we all must live, knowing all this effort is ultimately in vain. But until then, and if only for an evening, we are part of something greater; some engrossing event, in which our idiosyncrasies are one another's pleasure. Here, the host is able to 'kindle and illuminate', as Clarissa notes to herself. And later: 'how she had loved it all'.

There are Mrs Dalloways of fucking; hosts of arousal, climax, and their precarious moods. They are not all women, of course. See Daidd in SA Jones's *The Fortress*, knowing just how to suck Jonathon's cock. This is not just random tugging and slurping: the man knows his business. 'Daidd held Jonathon tightly around the base … with his thumb and forefinger, then pressed the head of his penis to the roof of his mouth and moved up and down the shaft, licking him.' Alas, this kind of precise sexual effort is so often feminised, and so dismissed as simple or easy. Think of the many labours of sex workers. Often involving specific hygiene and health requirements; specific clothing, like lingerie or fetish costumes; specific conversations, both fiscal and erotic; then the very physical work of tailoring sex to someone's taste — sex work is rarely just lying still.

It can also be a craft, which asks for sympathy and practical wisdom. Observe the planning that goes into music, considered an afterthought by some. Scientist and former call girl Brooke Magnanti recommends being sensitive to someone's musical tastes — including the possibility that their tastes are wrong. Having watched countless films with soft focus and soft soundtracks, maybe a lover believes they need schlocky love songs. But something else entirely will help them get off. 'Someone who pounds your arsehole to the beat of Stravinsky's *Rite of Spring*, on the other hand,' Magnanti writes, 'is clearly passionate about the music.'

Take this logic, and generalise it to fashion, cosmetics, perfume, lighting, bedlinen, to say nothing of verbal and bodily communication — sex can be enormously theatrical. This is 'theatre', not because lovemaking is always spectacular or overwhelming, but because the sexual mood is as much psychological and social as physiological. One person's relaxed, relaxing orgasm is another's expertise. It takes enormous effort to let a lover forget all the effort involved — and how much more for both lovers to forget.

So, here I bow to these Clarissas of all genders and sexualities: for maintaining these thin bubbles; for keeping King Shahriyar anxiously waiting for the story to continue.

Tiresias' Secret

On the Vagueness of Others Getting Off

Was it good for you?

Varieties of this question occur with maddening regularity. Was it? Was it, huh? Did you come? Are you *sure*? Obviously the answer matters. It shows how careful a lover has been, or how turned-on a beloved, or how erotic the atmosphere — or just how honest the relationship is.

Looking more closely, things are certainly more complicated, and perhaps more awkward. Regardless of whether the answer is 'oh, yes' or 'ugh, no' or somewhere between the two, it is possible that the response will be literally unthinkable. Not because of deceit, foolishness, or malice, but because sexual pleasure is idiosyncratic. We cannot understand one another's enjoyment.

To explore this ignorance further, let us turn to those sexually knowing beings: the Greek gods.

A Celebrated Harlot

The pagan deities enjoyed sex rampantly, and none more so than Zeus, king of the Olympians. He epitomised the dominant male: the priapic, relentless, brutal predator, from whom no goddess or mortal was safe. Often, Zeus was not so much a lover as a principle of lust and entitlement; he was patriarchy, anthropomorphised. But a lover he was nonetheless, including with his wife and sister, Hera. Despite their bickering and scheming, this couple were portrayed as avid bed-partners. One story: their wedding night lasted for three centuries. Another: Hera renewed her virginity every year, bathing in a sacred spring. Another: when Zeus made love to Hera on Mt Ida's peak, the earth sprouted turf and blossoms. From Alexander Pope's translation of the *Iliad*: 'Thick new-born violets a soft carpet spread,/ And clustering lotos swell'd the rising bed.' At the very least, Zeus was an emblem of rampant and rabid sexual adventure.

In a moment of typically petty bravado, Zeus once described himself as the loser in all this; the generous lover, giving and barely taking. And hidden within this myth is an intriguing idea about sexual pleasure, and our capacity to share it with others.

Tipsy on nectar one day, Zeus began to tease Hera. 'Of course,' he said, no doubt with a galling smirk, 'you women get far more pleasure out of love than men do.' This was another way of downplaying his cheating. If women, including Hera, enjoyed sex more than men, then really his wife had nothing to complain about. She got her rocks off with Zeus far more than he got from Metis, Themis, Eurynome, Mnemosyne (his aunt), Dione, Selene, Maia, Eris, Electra, Europa, Io, Danae, Isomoe,

Eurymedousa, Demeter, Persephone (his daughter with Demeter), Karme, Himalia, Niobe — and so on. This was a spectacularly smug way of amplifying his virility while muting his infidelity.

To score this cheap point, Zeus turned to Tiresias, a Theban with rare and special knowledge: Tiresias had once been a woman. And not just any woman. For seven years, he was 'a celebrated harlot', as Robert Graves put it in *The Greek Myths*.

As someone who had 'experienced love' as both sexes, Tiresias was supposedly able to confirm or deny Zeus's cruel quip. The Theban famously replied that, if pleasure were measured on a scale of zero to ten: women enjoyed nine, men one. In short: Zeus was right. In her rage, the queen of the gods blinded Tiresias. Zeus compensated him for his loss with the gift of prophecy, and a long life. It was his knowledge of lovemaking that set the scene for his later role as a legendary seer in the *Odyssey* and *Oedipus Rex*.

Clueless

There is a great deal packed into this mythic box: masculine entitlement and power fantasies; the supposed mystery of the feminine; an old association between wisdom and punishment; the cachet afforded by some ancient Greek courtesans; the philanderer's empty audacity.

But equally fascinating is the rarely noted premise: when it came to sexual pleasure, the king of the gods had no authority. Zeus was acknowledged as the most powerful of the Olympians. He punished criminals, wielded his lightning with brutality but fairness, watched over oaths and protected the sanctity of marriage (of

course he did). One of his epithets was 'wide-seeing' or
'all-seeing' — not quite omniscient, but close. And the
'panting thunderer', as Pope put it, was certainly no
stranger to love.

Yet Zeus's strength or bedpost notches were not
enough to put himself in his partners' sandals. He might
have said he knew Hera's pleasure — this was his gambit.
But he needed help from a lowly mortal to prove his
claim. For all his might, nous, and promiscuity, the god-
father was clueless. Zeus could assume, assert, speculate,
or simply take their word for it. But he could never know
his lovers' pleasure as he knew his own; he could never
rival Tiresias's first-hand knowledge.

Impenetrable Mysteries

This seems like merely a matter of physiology. Zeus might
have transformed into a swan or a shower of gold; might
have given birth to Athena — but he never became a
woman. (Why? This is another story.) Without a female
body, he could not put himself in even Hera's place, let
alone that of all women. And Europe has no monopoly
on this observation. 'Man and woman cannot know what
it is like in the other,' observes the *Kama Sutra*. Even if we
all seek orgasm, different flesh means different feelings.

This is to say nothing of gender — which is a cultural
phenomenon — alongside biological sex. The lustful
swaggerer, chasing the coy maiden; one to claim, the
other to be claimed. As Simone de Beauvoir catalogued
in *The Second Sex*, cultural tropes like these have long
characterised everything from flirting to orgasm — for
good or ill. Zeus, like so many men then and now, took

pleasure in possession; in control over another self. Put simply: he *took* pleasure. This, in turn, meant that his experience of sex and sexuality was at odds with most women's. In keeping with much of ancient Greek cosmology, he was a principle of activity, spirit — women, of passivity, matter.

Here, the king of the gods stands in for a common modern idea. Men cannot know women's pleasure, and vice versa, because they have different bodies *and* different social and psychological roles. As long as these variations exist, their sensations and perceptions will also be varied. At the very least, the myth of Zeus, Hera and Tiresias suggests this: intimacy between heterosexuals will always be curtailed. However close straight folk get in the bedroom, there will always be some distance between their delights.

Indeed, physiology puts distance even between those who toy with sex and gender in surprising ways. In Jordy Rosenberg's *Confessions of the Fox*, the chimeric Jack Shepperd grows a something between his legs. Not exactly a vulva. Not exactly a penis, but another sexual organ. And with this, he — the hero is a 'he' despite his ambiguity — fucks his lover, Bess Khan. And this fucking is novel to him as well as her. With his new something comes a lupine savagery alongside the tenderness; curious joining that threatens as much as it consoles. 'They made a hot Suture,' Rosenberg writes. 'A boiling Suture.' There is far more to the story than physicality, but the point stands: there are things we cannot know because we lack the special flesh to know them.

Yet this ignorance, ours and Zeus's, does not arise simply from erogenous zones or patriarchy. It is not simply about sex or gender, although these obviously guide experience. We cannot always comprehend others' pleasures because pleasure itself is highly personal; it has a keen first-person quality.

Take Zeus himself. Alongside his many female lovers (victims), the king of the pantheon had one notable male: Ganymede. The beautiful Trojan shepherd boy was abducted by Zeus — as an eagle this time — and taken to Olympus. There, he was cup-bearer, pouring wine-cups and bringing the monarch's sweet mead. But he was also Zeus's 'bedfellow', to use Graves' genteel word. This is important, because it allows us to consider Zeus, not as a stereotypical heterosexual patriarch, but as someone able to enjoy sexual pleasure with males and females, without shame. And in this capacity, he was *still* unable to fully understand his partners' pleasure.

Suppose Ganymede enjoyed being penetrated. Yes, this is troubling — the older, more powerful man and his powerless youth. There is no denying the patriarchal hierarchy here. But because Zeus was a divinity, he could force enjoyment upon the boy. The gods gave mortals immense and intense pleasure, whether they wanted it or not — whether they survived it or not. Witness the Homeric hymn to Aphrodite: 'a man does not enjoy vital vigor who goes to bed with immortal goddesses'. In contrast, Zeus would probably have found sodomy socially repugnant, as he was the *erastes* not the *eromenos*: the lover, not the loved. Being fucked this way made the man 'like a woman', as historian Anna Clark puts it.

And this is no ancient pagan quirk. Many men today avoid being penetrated anally. Witness Trevor in Ocean Vuong's *On Earth We're Briefly Gorgeous*: the macho redneck, who simply cannot take his lover's cock. 'I don't wanna feel like a girl. Like a bitch.' And for those who have no trouble with the stigma, there can still be too little payoff. It is just not their thing. A recent review of population data in *Sexual Health* by Australian public health researchers Wendy Heywood and Anthony Smith concluded simply: 'the available data suggest not all homosexually active men engage in anal sex'. In his memoir *Moab Is My Washpot*, comedian and author Stephen Fry phrased it with more panache: 'buggery is not at the end of the yellow brick road somewhere over the homosexual rainbow'.

The point is not that anal sex is somehow the great decider; the wall between delight and horror. It might equally have been smacking, dirty talk, or drag that distinguished Ganymede from Zeus. Kinks are many and varied — and rightly so. The point is that ignorance can arise between men and men, women and women, and those whose fluid genders avoid these frozen categories. It is not merely the stuff of heterosexuality or mainstream gender identity. Not even Tiresias could lift Zeus out of his unknowing.

Witness Vivaldo in James Baldwin's novel *Another Country*. About to sleep with his childhood friend Eric, he finds himself suddenly baffled by this other man. He has fucked men before, but always brutally: more a mark of power than tenderness or even lust. Now, he is aware of the fragile strangeness of Eric's existence — and his own:

> The male body was not mysterious, he had
> never thought about it at all, but it was the most
> impenetrable of mysteries now; and this wonder
> made him think of his own body, of its possibili-
> ties and its imminent and absolute decay, in a
> way that he had never thought of it before.

Eric's alien self makes Vivaldo's feel suddenly more foreign — and this deepens Vivaldo's experience. But Eric is no less alien for this. And this is two white American guys, who know each other well. Baldwin's story is full of lovers — black and white, queer and straight, working and middle class — who are intimate physically, but not psychologically.

So, even with exactly the same physiology and stimulation — improbable and perhaps impossible anyway — two lovers cannot always have the same gratification. We ought to do away with the idea that the same bits of flesh simply cause the same experience — or that bits of flesh simply cause experience *at all*. This is an error anthropologist Sara Johnsdotter calls, in the journal *Global Discourse*, 'genital determinism'. We also ought to do away with cultural determinism, which says that our ethnicity or class necessitates certain feelings.

Joy is highly idiosyncratic. However much we try to empathise with our partners, some delights are simply beyond us. This is not because we lack sympathy, but because we simply cannot perceive their pleasure *as* pleasure. It is alien to us.

Bats

Importantly, my point is not that sexual pleasure is always private: closed-in, and never available to others. We are not shut-ins. Much of our so-called 'inner life' is available 'out there': in the public world. We can talk about a common universe of things and happenings, and make sense. Instead, my point is that this world has a 'mineness' to it; a perspective that is not necessarily shared and shareable.

This is one of the arguments made by philosopher Thomas Nagel in his famous essay 'What is it like to be a bat?' Nagel noted that we might know everything about wing physics, echolocation and the nutrition of an insect diet, and still have no idea about how things are from the bat's point of view. This is not because the animal is mysterious or shy, but because bats have bat minds. And no scientific description of objective bat information will allow us to know the bat's subjectivity, because the only way to understand this is subjectively. 'If I try to imagine this, I am restricted to the resources of my own mind,' Nagel wrote, 'and those resources are inadequate to the task.'

Nagel was weighing in on the science of consciousness here: showing that it is not clear what such an endeavour might look like. How do we give an objective account of something that is, by definition, subjective? The problem is not facts in general — the problem is the fact of our first-person experience of facts.

Putting aside broader and more fraught debates in the philosophy of mind and neuroscience, Nagel's bat is immediately helpful on Zeus's love life and the question of sexual pleasure. It reminds us that, however well we might portray our arousal or orgasm, this means little to someone without our feelings. 'The only orgasm you can know and talk about in its entirety,' psychiatrist John Money observed, 'is your own.' And this can also change, with age, mood, or situation. Money wrote carefully about the psychology and physiology of climax, what he called 'the zenith of sexuoerotic experience'. Still, the renowned expert confessed that this apex of joy was 'solipsistic': a world unto itself.

So, the question 'Was it good for you?' can be answered
with a throaty 'yes!' without the lover understanding what
this means. We might believe lovemaking is good, and be
right — without knowing *how*.

Be Humble

Because of this, we also ought to avoid turning our
personal kinks into universal facts; transforming a
private pleasure, however ordinary, into some necessary
part of the human condition. In his *Eroticism*, the French
philosopher and novelist Georges Bataille wrote about
the thrill of sullying beauty. More specifically: the man's
thrill as he sullies a woman's beauty.

For Bataille, writing in the fifties, transgression of
taboos was essential for eroticism. And much of his thesis
is familiar. We cannot fuck whenever and wherever we
like — and certainly not whomever. We have workaday
duties, which ask for calm foresight and patience, as
against trembling lust. In sex, we overcome these normal
states of mind, and leave ourselves vulnerable: naked,
swollen, oozing or gushing. We feel more porous, shaky,
mercurial — like we are decaying with age or rotting
in death. The erotic, as Bataille put it, 'opens the way
to death'. The point is made with more than a pinch of
drama, but it makes sense.

What makes less sense is Bataille's idea that beauty
is needed for transgression. Men like beautiful women,
he argued, because they enjoy spoiling purity: first, by
revealing the vulva; second, by penetrating it. In this
way, a pretty face is joined to the 'hideous animal quality
of the sexual organs'. Men get off on this spoiling of

spiritual loveliness; this combination of the pleasing and the putrid.

The obvious problem with Bataille's theory is that it describes *some* men's kinks — men for whom genitals were filthy, ugly and stinking. No doubt there was, for them, some thrill in seeing a woman of grace and charm suddenly turn bestial. Some men today enjoy ejaculating on a woman's face for this very reason, and *some* of their partners feel similarly: they consent to this play of purity and stain. From a woman interviewed anonymously in *Cosmopolitan* magazine recently: 'It's a bit degrading, which is ... a turn-on for me.'

But for those who see pussies or cocks (or both) as simply alluring; who find penetration intimate but not gross; who treat cum as proof of care not domination — for those lovers, desire has no relationship to debasement. They experience the erotic without needing to spoil or be spoiled. From Anaïs Nin's diary, written in the early thirties: 'With a madonna face, I still swallow God and sperm, and my orgasm resembles a mystical climax.'

In fact, genitals evoke all kinds of feelings: they can be gorgeous, hilarious, sexy, sad. A penis might be Shakespeare's various swords, or poet Sharon Olds' gastropods in 'The Connoisseuse of Slugs'. A vagina might be a Spanish galleon in seventeenth century poetry, or scallops in Rita Dove's 'After Reading *Mickey in the Night Kitchen* for the Third Time Before Bed'. It might invite Rosenberg's laudatory pages about quim and its marvellous taste and scent: 'Sweet marshmallow and warm breath; saltwater threaded with Violet.' The glory of fucking does not depend on the union of divine faces and satanic groins. Some genitals are even — dare to believe it — prosaic.

In sex, pleasure is common — but not the *same* pleasure, or sources of pleasure. Unlike Bataille, we ought to be humble in our conclusions.

Pleasure Is a Beetle

So, even a good lay can be mired in ignorance. And yet: it can still be thrilling, fulfilling, often tender. This is because sex is less about journeying into someone's psyche, and more about learning a common language. To say that someone's fingertips give us pleasure is not to somehow hinge open our skulls and show our partners tingles or shivers. And our use of these words, like 'tingles' or 'shivers', did not begin by first looking at others' brains. In communicating, we learn from others' communications; we learn to associate certain public sights or sounds with certain feelings. We do not know what is felt by others — not like we know our own sensations and perceptions. (In fact, we do not 'know' them in the abstract sense. We *are* them.) But we do know what is shouted, whispered, shrugged, pointed. And, in this way, we are born and raised into language, and our sense of others' existence goes hand-in-hand with communication.

In his *Philosophical Investigations*, Austrian mathematician and philosopher Ludwig Wittgenstein asked us to consider a beetle in a box. Everyone has a box of their own, but no one can see into anyone else's package. Nonetheless, they chat happily and at length about their beetles. Of course, there may be no actual insects inside. There might be mice, votive figurines of Zeus, or nothing whatsoever. Still, folks talk about their 'beetles', and everyone gets the gist: they are happy or sad, excited or regretful, aroused or turned off. This might be absurd, but it makes sense. The thing in the box 'cancels out, whatever it is,' wrote Wittgenstein.

For Wittgenstein, the beetle was pain: usually considered the most straightforward and obvious of feelings. We cannot be wrong about it. Even so-called 'phantom pain' still hurts. And in this way, pain seems to be essential to communication: surely, at the very least, we can all perfectly understand one another's stings and aches? Wittgenstein's idea was that we do not have to understand — not with some profound empathy. We do not need to peek into the box to see the beetle; we do not need to feel others' pain to talk about it. The 'object drops out of consideration', as Wittgenstein put it, and the conversation continues regardless. The same is true of pleasure. Conversation about these feelings is more about the customs of language than about mystical fusion of personalities.

The point is not that we cannot share sexual experiences; that we exist as little pinholes of existential solitude. Nagel is right to suggest that, if we are all humans, bats, or beetles, we can all have some similar feelings. The point is that we do not have to feel the same thing to give one another pleasure. A sigh, a gyration, a yelp, a grimace, a chuckle — these all become part of our sexual language. We learn that an arched back often means slow down, and a quick exhalation means speed up. We learn that a certain smirk usually means a certain kind of penetration, and a glare not. We learn that open shutters, sunshine and clean sheets encourage delight and ant plagues do not. And then we learn it all over again, with a new lover; or with the same lover, in another mood or stage of life.

So, all over the world, there are gaps: between
spouses, couples, one-night lovers, polyamorists and
orgiasts. There is goodwill, lust, technical know-how,
and everything from mild contentment to overwhelming
thrill. And yet: we simply do not fully understand one
another. The Greeks were right to portray a powerful god
as clueless, but wrong to believe someone who had lived
as a man and a woman might know more. Ignorance is
built into the very stuff of consciousness. To be a sexual
being is to risk not knowing — never knowing. Tiresias's
real secret was that, man or woman or both, he was often
as clueless as we all are.

Just as importantly, this lack of knowledge does not
matter — not to sexual fulfilment, at least. Perhaps this
is annoying to romantics, who believe that screwing can
achieve perfect oneness with a beloved; that we might
fill ourselves with one another, like Iphimedeia with
Poseidon's waters (Apollodorus: 'she fell in love with
Poseidon, and went down to the sea again and again,
where she would scoop water from the waves ... and pour
it into her lap.') But this is a false fantasy; a promise that
can never be kept. Sexual intimacy is not a divine union,
but a conversation. And its feelings of togetherness arise
from the fluency of the dialogue — even when nothing is
said.

Choke Me

On the Tenderness of Rough Sex

F is beneath me.

I am inside her, and she me: this time, her tongue in my ear. 'No Diggity' plays, hopefully muffling our noises. There is a piano lesson happening ten feet away, and we want to be courteous if not modest.

Not long before, I read Clive Barker's *Imajica*, in which the hero Gentle fucks a shapeshifter, the mystif Pie Oh Pah. I no longer remember the story, but the vision of this coupling lingers. Gentle was wholly within Pie Oh Pah, 'balls and all'. Meanwhile, the mystif was filling the hero's lungs with his own breath. 'They were both entered in this exchange,' Barker wrote, 'and enterer'.

I too am gentle. Gentle, because F is smaller, weaker than I; gentle, because I am a tough black belt in karate and she is artistic; gentle, above all, because this is not simply penetration, but existential oneness. I am not some brute, you see. Not thumping away like a pasty, hairy hammer. This is not the sex I watch — late at night after watershed — in Eastern European movies. This is a grand supernatural joining, you see.

(Another vision from that era: Hokusai's 'Dream of the Fisherman's Wife', with the maiden filled pleasurably by two octopuses. She sucks and is sucked; the octopuses grip and are gripped. F and I are both maiden and octopus — but not creepy.)

F is beneath me.

She has already orgasmed, but has moved from exhaustion to arousal again. And why not? We are, after all, romantically united. The power of my adoration — soft, compassionate, perhaps even protective — makes her horny, you see.

As I approach my own climax; as my world shrinks infinitely to rutting and expands infinitely to love; as she and I move together to yet another proof of our perfection — in short, as we fuck in the most civilised way, F whispers in my ear: 'choke me.'

Sick

I do not understand. I want to understand, but how?

I cannot simply say 'pardon' or 'say again, dear' as F licks and I thrust. This is not a tutorial conversation, in which arguments are clarified before acceptance or rejection. Sex is a romantic matter; a matter of care, guided by spontaneity and knack. And, of course: love. (I do not celebrate these beliefs — I merely confess them.)

I continue, preferring silent fucking to distracting talk. This works for a minute or so. But, smirking, F eventually pushes my chest away, looks up into my eyes and says again: 'choke me'. Neither a command nor a plea — but certainly not a cautious query. *Do this thing for me. Please.*

F is beneath me — but only physically. She is no opponent in the dojo; no bully on the street, cracking open my cheek. She is my loved, loving equal. Why would I choke her?

A better question for the Damon in that bedroom — framed *Star Trek: Generations* poster on the wall, jar of condoms by the futon — was: why would *she want* me to choke her?

I ought not to put my vague feelings into full thoughts — this falsifies them. But my hunch, as F pulled my palm under her chin, was that she was somehow sick. Not in general; not as a human being. But in that moment, as she began coaxing my fingers around her throat, she was not well.

Hunger for Surrender

On that afternoon, F was a masochist.

Named for the author Leopold von Sacher-Masoch by nineteenth-century sexologist Richard von Krafft-Ebing, the word describes 'the wish to suffer pain and be subjected to force'. This is not for glory on the battlefield; not because of duty or honour. The masochist gets off on harm, or the threat of harm. Though clinical examples were scarce in his age, Krafft-Ebing was certain that 'feminine masochism' was common enough. 'Many young women,' he wrote in his *Psychopathia Sexualis*, 'like nothing better than to kneel before their husbands or lovers.' The tone of misogyny is false, but the observation is not.

To begin, note that masochism need not be an interest in pain. Pain is certainly part of the buzz for some, but violence alone can be enough. Sometimes stinging or throbbing is not felt straightforwardly *as* pain, or what gets someone off is the ferocity or danger behind the smacks or ties; the helplessness that comes with being thoroughly dominated. This is what American author Sallie Tisdale, in her essay 'Talk Dirty to Me', describes as 'a hunger for surrender'.

Putting aside Krafft-Ebbing's medical judgements — that masochism is a 'perversion' of ordinary dependency — the doctor was right about the popularity of the kink. A recent review of the literature in the *Journal of Sex Research* by Joseph Critelli and Jenny Bivona found that roughly a third to half of women report regular rape fantasies. A study in the same journal by Canadian criminologists Christian Joyal and Julie Carpentier found that almost one in five women not only fantasised about surrender, but also had tried to fuck masochistically.

My point is not to make slavery some essential female characteristic, as happens in philosopher John Norman's series of pulp novels. (*Vagabonds of Gor*: 'The mere sight of a slave whip is … enough to make her juice.') Norman's stories are patriarchal propaganda, which turn some women's sexual interests into universal sexual availability. The tropes are false, and easily inverted. As Zadie Smith observes in her short story 'Sentimental Education', we can equally think of seemingly masculine domination as a kind of feminine power ('I subsumed him in my anus … I took his flesh and totally nullified it'). This is also true for queer sex. The narrator in *On Earth We're Briefly Gorgeous* sees sucking cock as a kind of power: 'to be inside of pleasure, Trevor needed me. I had a choice, a craft ...' So, we cannot simply take up that hackneyed trope: the penetrated being is passive, weak, empty, and so on. My point is simply that masochism is quite literally ordinary.

That something is common does not make it good. We have the word 'normalise' for this very reason: it can make something unhealthy or unjust seem familiar and therefore safe. After all, research reveals that those into rough sex tend to watch videos of rough sex. Perhaps F was misled or misguided by erotica?

Ours was one of the last generations to try things in the bedroom *before* seeing them in pornography. The dog-eared, faded magazines we discovered never featured choking, and the closest we came to the internet was high-school hypertext classes. And even if F had been introduced to masochism by pornography — as many are today — this might equally have been liberating, not tyrannising. Put another way, normalising is only harmful if what is normalised does harm. (After centuries of stigma, going down was normalised in the late twentieth century. A boon for all.)

No doubt rough sex can combine with malice and brutality — especially with male abusers and female victims, where the gender roles come easily. Coercion can be subtle or overt, financial or physical. This is portrayed in Sally Rooney's novel *Normal People*, in which masochist Marianne has a series of cruel boyfriends: from the callous nonentity Jamie to the manipulative Swedish photographer Lukas. The problem is not Marianne's longing for domination, but her lovers' lack of care, or even basic ethics. Eventually, Marianne finally accepts Connell ('she was in his power'), who possesses her as she does him: with love.

What *Normal People* does not show is that, because of their codes and scripts, bondage and domination relationships can be far safer than 'vanilla' ones. A recent study in *Archives of Sexual Behaviour* by psychologist Shannon Martin and colleagues sorted rough sex seekers into two groups: those into sadomasochistic play, and those with 'victim blaming attitudes' and 'lower empathetic concern'. The former are more likely to fuck communicatively; to speak and heed safe words. The latter are more likely to become rapists. In short: sadomasochism is not shorthand for patriarchal cruelty.

Psychologically, sadomasochism seems benign at worst, and actually healthy at best. A small study by Pamela Connolly found those into rough screwing are no more anxious or depressed than the general population. Better still, bedroom submissives seem to enjoy themselves more than others. In their article for *The Journal of Sex Research*, Joyal and Carpentier concluded that masochists — and especially women — 'are the most satisfied, driven, and active sexually'. What might seem ugly or vile to others is obviously wonderful for many.

Perhaps masochists like F have 'eroticised oppression', as Sallie Tisdale paraphrases it in 'Talk Dirty to Me'? Have they simply turned inequalities and injustices into a kinky game? The problem with this idea is that it — ironically — does not take women seriously. 'What a misogynistic worldview this is,' Tisdale continues, 'that women who make such choices cannot be making free choices at all.' Yes, patriarchy is real. For many centuries, men as a class have benefited from violence against women as a class — and still do. But at its best, bondage and domination is a sexual performance, involving two or more free selves. They are not bullied or manipulated;

not beaten or bribed. They *want* to be choked, tied, or whipped, because this gets them wet or hard. Their kinks are not somehow beyond society, but nor are they simplistically within it. If they want, they can enjoy the sadomasochistic spectacle while thoroughly rejecting and resisting patriarchal reality.

Indeed, some turn to bondage and domination to work on trauma; to gain some power over their own flesh and psyche. Feminist scholar Corie Hammers writes about queer, lesbian and transgender rape survivors, performing their own assaults during sadomasochistic play. The idea is not simply to 'cure' trauma, as if rough sex were a tonic that offered forgetful happiness. The idea is to learn more about trauma, and perhaps learn how to live *with* it. 'These reenactments … loosened trauma's corporeal hold,' Hammers writes, 'which included a pervading and at times paralysing numbness.'

I cannot say F was seeking my grip for therapy; that our sex that afternoon was medicinal. But I can say this: I was wrong to think her sick or deviant. There was nothing pathological in her lust. If her 'choke me' shocked me, this was because of my naivety, not her perversion.

Fucked Harshly

It is one thing to see masochism from the outside, as it were; to check its correlations with psychopathology or well-being, and pronounce it dangerous or safe. It is quite another to look inside: to understand more fully the submissive's joy.

We cannot know one another's pleasures — not fully. Even those who share physiology and identity can be alien to one another: one gets off on a sucked this or squeezed that, the other grimaces at the thought. The beetle in the box is horny but hermetic. Still, we can understand better, if not fully; we can glimpse, peek, peer.

The most obvious fact of choking is hypoxia: the lack of oxygen. Did F want to get off on breathlessness? Certainly, what experts call hypoxyphilia is a common enough buzz.

Cutting off blood to the brain does lead to euphoria, which is why some use poppers before fucking: the amyl nitrate is a chemical asphyxiation.

But F did not need strangulation to achieve this high — she might have more easily just held her breath. This is a common way to encourage orgasm, as are panting and groaning. Psychiatrist Torsten Passie and colleagues, writing in the journal *Medical Hypotheses*, suggest that hyperventilation might bring on a 'sexual trance', by changing carbon dioxide levels in the blood. This no doubt overlooks a great many causes of pleasure — social and psychological — but the point is clear enough: we can get breathless or lightheaded without being choked.

What F wanted was not simply hypoxia; not simply some physiological reflex. She wanted to be fucked harshly, with my hands on her throat. This is why psychiatrist Stephen Hucker argues that the medical word for this kink ought to be 'asphyxiophilia' not 'hypoxyphilia'. 'These individuals,' Hucker writes in the journal *Archives of Sexual Behaviour*, 'primarily obtain sexual arousal by restricting their breathing, which secondarily results in the subjective experiences of oxygen lack.' And this restriction was one of being subservient, acquiescent. As a submissive, what turned F on that afternoon was the idea of domination.

The Palm of My Hand

For me, this was perhaps the most puzzling part of F's lust: not that she was seeking euphoria, but that she sought it in my violence. It was consensual violence, but violence nonetheless. She was no fighter, preferring Fauvism and jazz harmonies to my more lumpen karate. And even if she had been pugilistic, the bedroom was not the dojo or gymnasium — we fuck for tenderness, not truculence. Right?

At first blush, it does seem absurd to get horny about danger. Given how fragile and fleeting our moods are, being frightened seems a distraction. Arousal needs *just* the right state of mind to continue. And anything that changes our atmosphere, changes our erotic life.

Depression, for example, can weaken libido. Those who are depressed can sometimes screw and climax just fine, once they get going — but they do not want to. Studies regularly find that 'lack of positive affect' stops us from getting aroused. We need some spare change to be horny, and depression leaves us poor, like F. Scott Fitzgerald in 'The Crack-Up': 'for a long time I had not liked people and things, but only followed the rickety old pretence of liking.' Fitzgerald was not talking about sex, but his phrasing is apt: chronic stupor impoverishes our likes.

But while being choked, F was more likely to be afraid than anaesthetised. What does anxiety, or so-called 'negative affect', do to lust? For psychologists, anxiety comes in two main measures: 'trait' and 'state'. Those with high trait anxiety are prone to its symptoms more generally — part of their everyday life, alas. Others feel anxious in one state or another — it depends on the situation. As it happens, fear and horror have a complicated relationship to sex. Writing in the *Journal of Homosexuality*, psychologists Tera Beaber and Paul Werner report that straight women who suffer from more general anxiety often fail to climax while fucking. They get close, but lose it as feelings like guilt, anger, regret undo their mood. Lesbians are rarely troubled in the same way, interestingly — they have the angst *and* the orgasms.

And yet: not all fear or wariness is a turn-off. Instead of weakening concentration, a little state anxiety can actually strengthen it. In the journal *Behavior Research and Therapy*, psychologists Andrea Bradford and Cindy Meston suggest that fear primes the sympathetic nervous system, known to play a role in arousal. This does not always help with the subjective erotic mood — that is, with *feeling* horny. But it does help with vaginal tumescence and lubrication. And in Bradford and Meston's study, women who were jittery but not freaked out were physically *and* mentally titillated. From Roxane Gay's short story 'Bone Density': 'After he comes, in a loud, ugly display that always scares me in the way I like, my lover and I lie next to each other smoking.'

So, what horror aficionados have guessed for generations seems to be true: a good scare can get our blood up. This need not be from the stuff of fright-night: zombies, pin-headed freaks, clowns. Ordinary strife will do. Witness Naomi, from David Cronenberg's novel *Consumed*: 'She admitted to distracted sex, thinking about arguments she'd had with her mother or her sister, even ratcheting up the anger and intensity to the point of orgasm.' Granted, this is a very Cronenbergian vision — but this does not mean it is false. Think also of the anonymous woman in Anaïs Nin's short story, 'The Woman on the Dunes'. She tells her lover she once watched a Russian terrorist hanged in Paris. In the push of the crowd, a man presses up against her. Because she is so on-edge, she welcomes him. As the criminal on the scaffold falls and dies, the man behind her enters her then comes. 'She was palpitating with fear, and it was like the palpitation of desire,' Nin wrote. 'As the condemned man was flung into space and death, the penis gave a great leap inside of her, gushing out its warm life.'

In those moments before climax, we take whatever jolts we can. For F, the jolt was literally in the palm of my hand.

On Caring Less

Perhaps one consequence of F's arousal: I disappeared from her mind, if only briefly.

One of the ironies of sex is that the minutes of greatest physical and emotional intimacy can also be those of greatest solitude. Not because we feel sadly alone; not because of some grave alienation. It is because sometimes our awareness *must* shift from another self to our own. As more of our consciousness is given over to pleasure, the horizons of our world narrow. Or, to tweak the metaphor: our world ceases to be peopled by selves, and is instead populated by our own erotic sensations and half-thoughts.

When fucking, I believe F sometimes needed less of me, and more of herself. She loved me — I do not doubt this. But she was also chafed and rasped by my existence. The author James Bradley once said of me: 'I hear "Oliver's Army" play every time I see him.' Bradley's quip was not that I am a Cromwellian Roundhead or English imperialist. But the choice of music was apt, even if accidental. There is a force to my manner that can make even intimates uneasy or uncomfortable. (Andrew Marvell on Cromwell: 'thou, the war's and fortune's son,/ March indefatigably on;/ And for the last effect/ Still keep thy sword erect'.) Perhaps the force of my desire hindered F's pleasure.

If so, my choking of F might have made me *less* psychologically meddlesome for her. Research by Chinese neuroscientists showed that submissive rough sex players were less sensitive to others' emotions. In a recent paper for *Neuropsychologia*, Siyang Luo and Xiao Zhang observed that dominated women into sadomasochism were noticeably less empathetic. The same authors also note that ball-gagged masochists were especially dulled to others' feelings. In the journal *Frontiers in Neuroscience*, they speculate that the clamping of the submissives' faces and general humiliation worked together to make them more stony.

This finding from contemporary brain science nods to the ideas of philosophers like Friedrich Nietzsche, Merleau-Ponty and, more recently, George Lakoff and Mark Johnson. These thinkers argue that concepts cannot be understood dualistically: as if the mind were ethereal, floating away from the gross body. Our ideas are fleshy, visceral, muscular; arising from a physical world, and our physical dealings with it. We rely on our own corporeality to judge others' states of mind; we ape their flesh with our own, living our way into their experiences.

Because of this, throttled or bound masochists might find themselves less able to reach out to others — literally and figuratively. And this might be *exactly* what submissives need to get off. Instead of having another psyche forced upon them, they can revel in their own sexual selves.

In other words: perhaps F needed my hand to push me away — and thereby find herself.

No Small Thing

If F was retreating into herself, this was still happening within our relationship. However much her kink was new to me, F was asking me to preserve — and even develop — our couple-hood.

Allow me to entertain the thoughts I avoided, those many years ago.

To grip my girlfriend's throat; to press on the pale flesh there, as I had with a thug in a movie theatre; to stop her lifeblood as it moves from heart to brain; to tear capillaries and break skin — this is no small thing. This is decisive. As profound as the first kiss or fuck — perhaps more so, as it involves a wholly new intimacy.

Or does it? Much of this seemingly shocking novelty was already part of our love.

Sadomasochism begins and ends with respect, or it is merely assault. There can be no coercion; not even sneaky passive-aggressive sulking. It must be freely consented to, or it is abuse. Witness the world of seventies San Francisco gay sadomasochism, documented in Edmund White's *States of Desire*. At first, this might seem one of terrifying machismo — all that leather, steel, and testosterone. But despite the semblance of savage male violence, the games of bondage and domination were civilised. They had their rituals of communication and consent; their special signs and symbols. 'The freedom to start and stop a sex scene,' White wrote, 'is part of almost every S&M contract.' And witness that word, 'contract': this is the formal language of those who know the terms must be unambiguous, unprejudiced.

F and I were already in this milieu of care and honesty. We had negotiated virginity and threesomes; had dealt with stomach bugs and anxiety, rightful jealousy and pointless paranoia; had continuously, sometimes annoyingly *talked*. In short, there was little to surprise us in the rites of rough sex.

Harm is also part of every romance. Not because of strangulation, but because love itself is a risk. We commit ourselves to another human being, who is as changeable as we are.

They might cheat on us. They might age out of their libido, and leave us mad with lust. They might become bitter, or we might become jaded. Whatever the span of the affair — from days to decades — there are enough moments for us to fail one another. And there is no other way to love. As Nussbaum puts it, love is a 'relational good'. To enjoy its benefits, we have to put up with its inconstancies and instabilities. Even if we miraculously avoid hurting one another with profound betrayal or a thousand petty cruelties, there is always mortality. 'Grief,' Nussbaum writes in *The Fragility of Goodness*, '… becomes a natural part of the best human life'. We cannot help harming those we live alongside, if only because we will one day stop living altogether.

There was — and still is — goodwill between F and me. But we were always going to hurt one another — somehow. In this, choking was the muscular face of a more general spectre. A spectre we welcomed, because romance depends on this haunting.

Also, F's kink was part of her psyche already. Perhaps she had only just recognised its force. Perhaps she was worried about revealing it. But the need — to get off on being brutalised — was obviously an important one. My point is not that she was somehow fated to be a gasper, or that she still is. Her lusts today are none of my business. My point is simply that sexual tastes are deep and strong, and they cannot be shrugged away. In fact, they *ought* not be shrugged away — it is psychologically dangerous to deny healthy sexuality.

So, choking F was not as novel as it seemed at the time. We were already a trusting couple, familiar with love's threats. And F was already someone who longed to be roughly taken, if only briefly. In this light, we were not tip-toeing on thoroughly alien soil.

And yet, and yet ...

My hunch was right nonetheless: choking a lover is no small thing. This is deliberate physical brutality, rather than accidental grief or regret. It is the confession of a stigmatised kink, rather than simply a preference for, say, hirsute dudes. (What philosopher Robin Dembroff calls a 'druther', as in 'I'*d rather* thick black hair than smooth skin.') However much a sadomasochistic relationship was familiar to me, knowingly manhandling F was both foreign and very serious. Our love would change.

But how?

Masters and Slaves

The first change was one of savagery. To dominate F in this way, I had to confront my own violence.

There can be a frenzy to sex; a feeling that these forces are welling up without concern for propriety, let alone love. Necessity is familiar to most of us: the sense that arousal and orgasm *must* be. And violence can have this same feeling. Think of the ancient berserkers, who were overwhelmed by their own bloodlust during battles. They 'raged uncontrollably in a trance of fury,' writes historian Michael Speidel. Naked, without armour, they kept killing until all their foes were dead — or they were.

In sadomasochism, these two necessities fuse: aggression and lust. 'When your blood's up,' says George in DH Lawrence's *The White Peacock*, 'you don't hang half way.' He is speaking of hunting rabbits, but also about fucking. Witness Rufus in James Baldwin's *Another Country*, ejaculating his 'venom' into poor, much-abused Leona. '*I told you*, he moaned, *I'd give you something to cry about*.' As I balanced on that futon with F, did I really want to give in to this barbarity? This was a complicated choice, to say the least. As the child of a violent home, I had no wish to continue men's violence against women; no wish to justify bruises with my madness. Strangulation was for male enemies, not female lovers.

Put another way, to choke F was to make *both* of us vulnerable. She was threatened by my grip, but I was also threatened: by the loss of myself. I was naked, without armour.

The second change was between master and slave. At first blush, it all seemed simple. As a submissive, F was an object of sorts; something to whom things were done by me, the subject. I was the scary strong man, she the frightened weak woman. But sadomasochism often transcends such tropes. 'A real sadist does not want the other person's consent,' says French dominatrix Catherine Robbe-Grillet, 'a real sadist does not want the other person's pleasure.' To strangle F sexily but safely, I must be caring, patient, observant — in a word: attentive. I must devote myself to the techniques of arousal; to the precise rhythms and pressures that get her off. 'The top needs to hurt the bottom,' Finnish philosopher Timo Airaksinen writes his essay 'A Philosophical and Rhetorical Theory of BDSM', 'and at the same time recognise and serve her, otherwise he is not a good top.' By asking to be choked, F asked me to submit to *her* domination.

F is beneath me — and I must stoop to serve her. I must crouch, and make myself smaller.

No

By asking me to choke her, F also invited me to better myself.

She asked me to witness her seemingly alien kink; the frenzied needs behind her calm persona. She asked me to think more about the quirks that turn fear into lust; that transform instincts of flight into those of fucking. She asked me to be humble; to allow myself to grow smaller in her perception, and as a master who served. She asked me to be more solicitous, perhaps even reverential; to learn these techniques of patient ardour. And above all, she asked me to mature as a man; to live with seemingly conflicted passions and roles, and perhaps even enjoy this strife. She asked me to join her in a more nuanced adulthood.

She asked, and I answered 'no'.

I did not choke her. I never choked her.

Solomon Kane's Demon

On Beauty and Politics

Tall, lean, and corpse-pale, Solomon Kane is riding across the Carpathian mountains when he sees her: a pagan statue of a woman. She is wearing a halterneck, and little else: two strips of fabric crossed over her nipples, a simple loincloth, and a skullcap over her straight blonde hair.

Does he stand and gape? Does he bow chivalrously? Does he perhaps sketch her?

Nay. The hero steps back and raises his palm to ward her away. He knows she is but marble, the work of some sculptor centuries before. Yet he feels possessed by her — and now he wants to possess her in turn. He monologues to himself, clenching his fists. Then he screams, praying to his God: 'give me the strength to resist all impure desires'. The adventurer topples the statue, smashing her on the temple stones.

Grateful the danger is gone, Kane celebrates his gift to the world's innocents. 'It is done, heavenly lord! That which momentarily bewitched me,' he says to the rubble, 'shall no longer bewitch anyone, especially one of a weaker will!'

Blade of Righteousness

So begins the comic 'The Cold Hands of Death', published in *The Savage Sword of Conan* in 1977. It was written by Don Glut, though Kane was invented by Texan author Robert E. Howard in the late twenties.

Kane is notable for his dour austerity. While his literary brother Conan the barbarian drinks and screws, the Englishman broods in chaste sobriety. In his narrow Puritan psyche, there is room only for a little lust: martial, not erotic. Kane is fine with lead spattering brains; with steel puncturing lungs. More than fine: the pulp hero is often exhilarated by violence. 'It was with a certain ferocious fascination that he faced his howling attackers,' Howard wrote in 'The Footfalls Within'. 'The flickering rapier parried the whistling scimitars and the Arab died on its point, which seemed to hesitate in his heart only an instant before it pierced the brain of a sword-wielding warrior.'

So killing is fine, but fucking? Not on his life. (Quite literally. When offered freedom and conquest to wed and bed a queen, the Englishman shuns her.) While he once had a lover in his Devon village, Kane has now sworn off love and lovemaking alike. He has many close relationships with the men he kills — thrusting, gripping, and gazing without blinking. And he abandons himself to these without pause. But the statue of a gorgeous woman, standing before him in thin linen? Suddenly, the hero is gnashing and foaming with doubt — she must be destroyed. Having vanquished the temptation, Kane retires to an inn and believes himself safe. But the woman returns in his dreams, standing in front of his bed: 'her flawless body,' wrote Don Glut, 'radiant as marble kissed by the setting sun'. Kane tries to resist, but his will is weaker in sleep's fantasy. They fuck. And suddenly the Puritan feels his strength going; feels like he felt on the battlefield, 'his blood spilling a crimson stream'. This ancient heathen is a demon; a succubus, who steals his great energies for herself. He can only defeat her by rejecting her enchantment, which he finally does with the help of a broken old mirror. He sees her face for what it really is: somewhere between a fish, a lizard, and a lion. He lifts his 'blade of righteousness', and cuts off her head.

The danger is gone.

Succubus

Perhaps this story is bizarre to readers of modern literary fiction; perhaps they see this as little more than pulp fantasy. But these are ancient and ubiquitous sexual tropes.

The succubus was a popular spectre in medieval Europe. From the Latin for 'lying beneath', succubi were supposedly the spawn of Lilith, a Babylonian demon. Stories about Lilith occurred throughout Mesopotamia, and she was also the desert bird that haunted the prophet Isaiah: 'the screech owl also shall rest there, and find for herself a place of rest'. Similar villains existed in folklore across the world, arising partly from what psychiatrist Sandeep Grover and colleagues call 'sleep paralysis and hypnagogic hallucination'. Finding ourselves limp and numb in the middle of the night, we invent monsters 'out there' to take the blame, instead of our own physiology 'in here'. And we do so from within our own cultures, so these monsters are often patriarchal caricatures: sultry vampires, who harm naive men with their own ardour. The *Zohar*, a medieval Jewish text, says:

> [w]herever these spirits find people sleeping alone
> in a house, they hover over them, lay hold of
> them and cleave to them, inspire desire in them
> and beget from them. They further inflict disease
> on them without their being aware ...

In this, the succubus is a perfect enemy for Solomon Kane. She evokes the terror of paralysis, a common feature of heroism — especially for the tense, restless Puritan, used to wandering wherever he chooses. More importantly, she adds lust to this drama. Kane must struggle to overcome, not only feebleness, but also horniness. 'No matter how he attempts to fight the temptation,' wrote Glut, 'he becomes its slave.' Warriors can be killed with a quick lunge or strong punch. But this blonde demon? Kane can only defeat her by first conquering his own manhood. So, the succubus is an existential test, which Kane passes with pious discipline — and, more importantly, with good luck. Ultimately, he prevails because he witnesses her hidden physiognomy; her nauseating face. Kane knows she is a predator, and he her prey. He knows he is being fucked to death in his bed. Nothing changes in his fear or fury. What changes is only the demon's looks: in that glass, 'he beholds the true form of the hellish "beauty" in whose embrace he is locked'.

The succubus fails and dies because she is ugly.

And yet: the succubus never really loses her beauty. As drawn by penciller Steve Gan, she is briefly hideous before Kane chops at her neck — but the stone head he finally throws to the ground is gorgeous.

As is another succubus, whom Kane meets in Howard's tale 'The Moon of Skulls'. This ancient villain is a fiend for men's blood — that is, their life force. And, like her blonde ancestor, she is beautiful but evil. 'She is Lilith — that foul, lovely woman of ancient legend.' It is this queen Nakari who offers Kane a kingdom for marriage, an offer he is briefly enchanted by. He dreams of uniting Europe with force, but he is also drawn to Nakari's exotic looks. She is 'naked except for a beplumed helmet, armbands, anklets and a girdle of coloured ostrich feathers,' Howard wrote. And she is not simply pretty, but 'regal yet barbaric, haughty and imperious, yet sensual, and with a touch of ruthless cruelty about the curl of full red lips'.

So, two vampiric women: both deadly, and both gorgeous. And they *must* be gorgeous, because only beauty is a danger to the Puritan's soul.

Why? Because beauty makes *him* ugly.

Ezigbo Mmada

Like many pious souls, Solomon Kane is wary of physical beauty, because he seeks a higher beauty: that of the self.

The Igbo of West Africa have a phrase for this: *ezigbo mmada*. In classical Igbo culture, this means someone good. A stalwart of their family, tribe and town, they exemplify common values. They are caring, generous, respectful of the gods and ancestors — what Nigerian philosopher Christopher Agulanna describes in the *Journal of Pan African Studies* as 'one who sets things right in the community'.

For the Igbo, this ethical character is beautiful. Humanity is not merely another animal; another bag of meat and bones, to eat or be eaten. We are the pinnacle of divine creation, and our behaviour ought to continue this godly splendour. Anthropologist Chinyere Ukpokolo argues that, in this worldview, Igbo individuals are responsible for keeping their souls comely. 'One can lose the beauty that the Supreme Being/God has bestowed on him or her,' she writes, 'hence the need to nurture and protect it.'

Here, it is not enough to be pretty. This is obviously sought after, but it cannot guarantee beauty in the community. This is because beauty exists only in context: this value, that belief, these rites, those gestures. 'Experience of beauty has to do with wholeness and interdependence,' notes philosopher Diana-Abasi Ibanga in her paper 'The Concept of Beauty in African Philosophy', 'and recognising one's place in the connective web of other existents.' There is no essence of beauty, passed along from face to face. It must be lived, and always among others.

Importantly, one of the chief virtues of this beautiful soul is calm: a good self cannot be manic or mad. While the *ezigbo mmada* defends community harmony, they cannot merely be the individual containers for communal spirit; cannot be porous, constantly soaking up everyone's passions. They must be, as Agulanna puts it, 'level-headed, imperturbable or unflustered'.

Interestingly, some art traditions from Africa involve similar ideas of equipoise. The Yoruba people speak of *àsà*, which can be translated as style: a distinct way of doing things. And this 'way' refers to broader traditions, as well as the artists working within these traditions. To develop the most beautiful *àsà*, the sculptor or painter must be calm. This allows them to be in touch with the ancestors, as well as with the *ìwà*, or essence, of themselves and their work. In his paper 'African Aesthetics' in *The Journal of Aesthetic Education*, art historian Rowland Abiodun observes that the good creator must have 'gentle character ... as well as patience ... poise ... grace,' and sums this up with a single word: 'cool'. This is not simply being fashionably aloof or ironic. Like the Igbo *ezigbo mmada*, the cool Yoruba artist is divine. 'To act in foolish anger or petty selfishness,' writes historian Robert Farris Thompson, 'is to depart from [the] original gift of interiorised nobility and conscience.' Put another way: to make beauty, I need a beautiful self.

Psychological beauty is also required to recognise it in others. Yes, I can be carried away by sculpture or music — what philosopher Justin C. Njiofor calls its 'power to refresh, enliven, energise, and uplift'. But art is no excuse for mental caprice or laziness. A true critic is carefully, slowly cultivated. They develop only after years of education, learning from the community elders. And to even begin this, the budding critic has to have sensitivity, constancy, perseverance, and *ìfarabale*: what Abiodun translates as 'calmness and control'. Transcending mere looks, the cool observer is able to see the moral goodness beneath the pleasing shapes and colours. In doing so, they are connected to 'the linchpin wheel of the African ethical system', as Njiofor puts it in 'The Concept of Beauty'. To see grace and charm, I need a graceful and charming soul — and one that remains so, aloof and serene.

In this light, ugliness is more than plainness or clumsiness. It is a sign of vice. The cowardly, hasty or brutal soul is hideous. Like Solomon Kane's various vampires, they might indeed be pretty or hot. But they themselves are actually gross: distorted, distasteful selves, who can neither create nor appreciate true beauty.

In this mythos, the succubus is dangerous because her beauty makes men stupid or mad; makes their minds dulled or muddled. When Solomon Kane cannot help fucking the demon, he becomes demonic in turn. His physique is still athletic; his sword arm still swift, fists still hard; his eyes still 'mystical deep pools that drowned unearthly things'. But his psyche is weak and mad. He is no longer an *ezigbo mmada* — he cannot set things right in the community. He cannot even set himself right. Beauty has made the hero ugly.

Four-Footed Beast

Neither American pulp nor African philosophy have a monopoly on this wariness of good looks; this anxiety that another's beauty can spoil our own.

At the very beginnings of Greek thought and literature we see the same worry: that erotic beauty is a thief, robbing us of equipoise. The poet Sappho called Eros a 'limb-loosener', while Anakreon a generation later described the same god as a blacksmith, knocking him into a ditch with an enormous hammer. In *Sophist*, Plato wrote of the good soul as harmonious, and foolishness as 'deformed and devoid of symmetry' — in a word, ugly.

Elsewhere, he described *eros* as a kind of madness, which pulls the psyche away from beautiful goodness, towards the muck and mire of screwing. In *Phaedrus*, the philosopher eventually recognised the ethical value of longing: the lover seeing the transcendent Forms in his beloved's form. But this had to be chaste. Anyone still interested in fucking ends up 'surrendering to pleasure,' he wrote, 'after the fashion of a four-footed beast'.

So, the Greeks celebrated beauty's pull on us, but also lamented the violence and cruelty of this wrenching. 'Eros is an enemy,' writes poet and classicist Anne Carson in *Eros the Bittersweet*. 'Its bitterness must be the taste of enmity. That would be hate.' Nineteenth century Irish poet Thomas Moore was less melodramatic than these Hellenes, but equally sure of beauty's power to undo reason and dignity: 'Though Wisdom oft has sought me,/ I scorn'd the lore she brought me,/ My only books/ Were woman's looks,/ And folly's all they've taught me.'

This might seem like a poetic or scholarly conceit: exaggerating beauty out of romantic tension or numbed repression — and certainly Sappho and Plato suggest these at times. Not all eros leaves us 'frantic-mad with evermore unrest', as Shakespeare put it. Not every smitten lover is, as Renaissance poet Petrarch described, like a butterfly flying towards the sun to its death. But as a species, *Homo sapiens* is profoundly sensitive to beauty. While this beauty is varied and shifting — changing within lives, eras, and civilisations — what it does to us is remarkably reliable.

Scientists divide the sexual brain into three systems: attraction, consummation, and attachment. These describe coming together, screwing, and staying together, and fit well with Irving Singer's categories of eros, libido, and romance. Beauty is especially important to the first of these, the erotic: when someone first stands forth to me. This is the moment when Leonard Woolf saw the sisters Vanessa and Virginia Stephen, with their white dresses and parasols. 'One stopped astonished,' he wrote in *Sowing*, 'and everything including one's breathing for one second also stopped'. (Reader, he married Virginia just over a decade later.) Importantly, attraction need not always lead to adoration, which turns a specific someone into a target, and me into a loosed arrow. This is what anthropologist Helen Fisher and colleagues, in their paper 'Romantic Love', describe as an evolutionary adaptation for 'conserving courtship time and metabolic energy'. Beauty is simply the beginning of this possible brain change, involving a release of dopamine and a sudden interest in one person to the exclusion of others. While this neurotransmitter can make me single-minded, it can also leave me 'giddy', as Fisher observes elsewhere. Here, I am suddenly clear about who I want, but not necessarily about anything else. From Romantic poet John Clare's 'First Love': 'My face turned pale as deadly pale,/ My legs refused to walk away,/ And when she looked, what could I ail?/ My life and all seemed turned to clay.'

So, unless I am intimidated, beauty is typically gratifying — whether I like it or not. If I am in a good mood, Fisher reports, seeing someone pretty or sexy actually lowers my cortisol levels, leaving me less anxious. To encounter someone pretty or handsome is to find myself inadvertently and involuntarily changed. And if I regret my paled cheeks or empty lungs later, this does not stop me coming back for more. I keep up Petrarch's flight, Clare's jelly legs, or Solomon Kane's faint.

Pretty Capital

The beautiful are typically rewarded for these primal gifts.

Witness: teachers often see pretty children as smarter, and more likely to achieve high marks. Analysing several studies of primary and secondary schools, psychologist Vicki Ritts and colleagues observe bluntly: 'highly physically attractive students ... are the beneficiaries of more favorable judgments by teachers.' Importantly, these kids often *do* achieve better grades, though there is a weak correlation between beauty and the virtues that encourage academic success, like intelligence and conscientiousness. More likely is that beautiful children are expected, encouraged and supported to succeed — and they eventually take their own talents for granted. 'We are "blinded by beauty",' write psychologist Sean Talamas and others, concluding that these kinds of expectations can have 'alarming' consequences for pupils' education.

When they enter the workforce, the good-looking candidates are more likely to be called back for a job interview; more likely to be hired; more likely to receive higher pay; more likely to be promoted. They are also more likely to have prestigious jobs than their more plain or ugly peers, and this applies for entry candidates as much as for senior employees, according to preliminary research by sociologist Emanuela Sala and colleagues. A review of over twenty studies by psychologist Megumi Hosoda in the journal *Personnel Psychology* put it bluntly: 'physical attractiveness is always an asset for individuals'. In this way, the beautiful gain the benefits of wealth and high status. Because beauty is a performance and not simply a physiological gift, these allow them to bolster their quality of life *and* their comeliness: they can pay more for medicine, fitness, clothing, cosmetics, and surgery.

Pretty or handsome people can also form useful cliques, which offer them opportunities or support when needed. They do not simply have lots of friends and acquaintances, they manage and manipulate these to advantage — they have what management scholars Kathleen O'Connor and Eric Gladstone call 'broker positions in networks'. Because of their greater confidence and security, the beautiful can also take more risks.

Even before we get to lust and love, the beautiful have clout. They gain more cash, command and repute than others — more power, in other words.

The French sociologist Pierre Bourdieu wrote of power as 'capital', and divided it into kinds: economic, political, social, cultural. Perhaps the most well-known (and most popularly muddled) of these is social capital, which refers to cliques. In *An Invitation to Reflexive Sociology*, Bourdieu describes these as lasting webs of 'more or less institutionalised relationships of mutual acquaintance and recognition'. But the other forms of capital are equally important in Bourdieu's theory, describing the ways we gain and grow authority: through home life, schooling, friendships, employment, leisure. This is rarely done knowingly. Instead, we are 'born into the game, with the game', as he put it in *The Logic of Practice*. We learn very specific ways of thinking about the world and one another, but also ways of speaking, walking, dressing, eating — and no doubt flirting and fucking.

Sociologist Catherine Hakim refers to this as 'erotic capital', though her theory emphasises women's possession of this power — rather than men's continuing and often cruel possession of women. If capital is women's reward for playing the game well, this sport was invented, refereed, and sponsored by men.

So, while men have generally been the heirs of all forms of capital, beauty works for both genders. And it does so despite our smarts. The point is not that we are always foolish to reward beauty, but that we often do so unconsciously and unreasonably. Even if there are rational reasons to see beauty as hale and gainful — and these are complex judgements — we do not behave rationally. We have an immediate and intuitive reaction to someone's good looks, and this regularly overcomes our intellect. It is more a lurch and a hunch than a choice.

And this is why physical beauty is such a threat to Solomon Kane, and the ideal described by *ezigbo mmada*. I cannot necessarily be calm and disciplined; cannot think carefully of the greater good; cannot be cool. My existential beauty meets a gorgeous face or stunning body, and becomes demonic.

The Other

There is no denying beauty's psychological and social power; no avoiding the fact that comeliness in others undoes comeliness within ourselves.

More dubious, though, is who gets blamed for this — and how. In 'The Cold Hands of Death', Solomon Kane is a victim then victor. The succubus becomes a symbol of Solomon Kane's psyche — she stands in for his existential drama. Because of this, she is not a full self, with her own adventures; not a fellow traveller. The demon is a living sign of the Puritan's susceptibility to corruption. And she must be killed, to kill his own weakness.

Here, the woman is what Simone de Beauvoir, in *The Second Sex*, calls the Other. 'In every sexual act the Other is implicated; and the Other most often wears the visage of woman,' she wrote. 'Woman is vampire, she eats and drinks him.' As Other, this woman is not a whole human being. Instead, she is a tiny fragment of man's humanity. And because of this, her beauty is ultimately not her own: good or ill, it belongs to man, and is merely an enticement or a warning in his great adventure.

Suppose we asked the Other? She might rightly reply that beauty is often made painful by men's supposed entitlement to it. This Other could be Eva from Gabriel García Márquez's story 'Eva is Inside Her Cat', who wants to be finally rid of her own beauty. She is exhausted by it, 'tired of ... being under siege from men's long looks.' She could be eleven-year-old Lou from Lucia Berlin's 'Sex Appeal', whose cousin wants to date a rich boy. But the rich boy prefers Lou. 'He picked his lighter up and told me I had Baked Alaska on my chin. When he wiped it with the big linen napkin his arm brushed my chest.' She could be Ladydi from Jennifer Clement's novel *Prayers for the Stolen*, whose mother tries to make her look like an ugly boy. If she is a pretty girl, the Mexican cartels might kidnap her as a slave. 'Maybe I need to knock out your teeth, my mother said.' She could be Gillian from AS Byatt's tale 'The Djinn in the Nightingale's Eye', who is groped by her friend's father as he serves her breakfast. He pulls down her nightdress, holds her breasts, then 'snuffles' between them, saying he cannot bear her beauty. 'And I felt sick,' she remembers decades later, 'and felt my body was to blame.' She could be the Trojan princess Briseis in Pat Barker's novel *The Silence of the Girls*, taken as a prize by Achilles. The killer holds her chin, turns it to and fro like a horse's head inspected by a buyer. 'Cheers, lads,' says Achilles. 'She'll do.' And so on.

But the Other is not there to speak. Or, rather: she might flirt or whisper soothing words, but she is not there for conversation. Beauties are typically objects, not subjects. The right of reply belongs to those historical exemplars of public maturity: men. Which is why, in this worldview, women ought to be modest — preferably locked away privately in the kitchen or boudoir. This is needed to protect men from women's wiles, and to protect women from the consequences of their wiles. In either case, men will decide what ought to happen, and why. Yes, women might have Hakim's 'erotic capital'; might have swaying hips or red lips that 'bewitch anyone … of a weaker will.' But this wealth has rarely been fungible; rarely been convertible into economic, political, or educational assets.

And when beauty threatens — or threatens to threaten — men's assets with irrationality or incapacity? For the sake of Kane's emancipation, the succubus must be punished or killed.

The Drums

Likewise for Africa. In the Solomon Kane stories, it exists as an Other. In one of those painful colonial ironies, there is no *ezigbo mmada* among Robert E. Howard's Africans. The continent is written chiefly to provide savages to kill, simpletons to save — and symbols for Kane's moral conflict.

In 'Red Shadows', the Puritan travels to the jungles to kill a French brigand, Le Loup, or 'The Wolf'. Why?

Because the Wolf murdered a girl. She was a stranger to Kane, but her death was enough — Kane is forever wandering in search of righteous battle. Howard described his hero as 'a strange blending of Puritan and Cavalier, with a touch of the ancient philosopher, and more than a touch of the pagan'. In other words, Kane is by no means wholly rational or wholly Christian. He is a god-fearing killer — but a killer nonetheless.

In Howard's fantasies, Africa is a symbol of these atavistic urges, and others. It is there that Kane meets the vampire queen Nakari, and is tempted by glory and exotic beauty. 'The drums roared and bellowed to Kane as he worked his way through the forest,' Howard wrote. 'Somewhere in his soul a responsive chord was smitten and answered. You too are of the night (sang the drums); there is the strength of darkness, the strength of the primitive in you'. Yes, the civilised white Christian has primal urges — but Africans are shorthand for these.

Robert E. Howard was a racist, who believed most peoples of colour were straightforwardly lesser than whites. There is no denying or trivialising this. Howard wrote to fellow *Weird Tales* author (and nasty xenophobe) HP Lovecraft, 'I agree with you in doubting that the seeds of cultural development are present in the negroid race as a whole.' Nobody even fleetingly familiar with America's history will see Africa as more savage than Howard's white Christian Texas; than the colonials, with their slaves and genocide. Howard himself saw his 'Aryan' forebears as brutes. But they were *his* brutes, and he praised their conquering spirit. He was proud of his ancestors' murdering, pillaging, and exploitation of Africans. He contrasted their tough pioneering spirit with the supposed seedy cynicism of the 'Jew, Polack or Wop, spawned in some teeming ghetto', and said he longed to return to the old plantation era. In this way, whites like Howard fantasised about the 'lesser races' to glorify their own common greed and brutality. And a large part of this mythos was the mysterious dark continent, with its inscrutable and illogical ways.

As Nigerian novelist Chinua Achebe observed in his essay 'An Image of Africa', the whole continent is thereby turned into a European fantasy. There are no human beings in the jungle or village, just avatars of the *real* human beings: men like Solomon Kane. In the Kane tales, as in Joseph Conrad's *Heart of Darkness*, Africa becomes 'a metaphysical battlefield devoid of all recognisable humanity, into which the wandering European enters at his peril'.

And the African woman? She, too, is entered by Europeans at their peril. Not by Kane, of course. But as Queen Nakari, she is there for Howard's readers, with her 'young and … tigerish comeliness'. And she is in every colonial trope about savage, sexual blacks.

Historically, this trope continued with slavery, as white men sought to distinguish between their wives and their property. In America, country of upright, undefiled Christians, 'black women were naturally seen as the embodiment of female evil and sexual lust,' bell hooks wrote in *Ain't I a Woman*. 'They were labeled jezebels and sexual temptresses and accused of leading white men away from spiritual purity into sin.' This trope continues today for African American women and girls as the 'Jezebel' persona, a stereotype that minimises their humanity while maximising their sexuality. They are seen as, in the words of psychologist Danice L. Brown and colleagues, 'oversexed, promiscuous, angry and loud'. Puritan, beware.

These are all versions of the same white male story. In Africa, beauty is another enemy to be conquered for Solomon Kane's glory — lest he become spiritually ugly. There are beautiful dark women to conquer, and beautiful light women to save, all to keep our hero morally comely.

Cool Socrates

Yes, Solomon Kane is a fiction, and pulp fiction at that. And his macho chastity is as rare in literature as it is in life: manliness and horniness typically go together. But his adventures with the succubus, and in Africa, are suggestive. They show how erotic beauty becomes more than merely a superficial gift; more than the femme fatale's dark skin and dark eyes, or the innocent maiden's 'reddish gold hair ... fine grey eyes'. It is even more than a well-practiced swagger or smirk. Instead, it is a lived moral category, used to maintain a social hierarchy: ideal truth or physical falsehood; masculine dignity or feminine curse; pure white shield or tainted black weapon.

Beauty might *feel* simple: from weak knees, to a vague sense of talent or virtue, to something like a personal welcome. But it exists within a complex cultural order. And this order is often indifferent to justice, and almost always insidious — I am playing Bourdieu's game before I realise it is a game (if I ever do).

The real demon of Solomon Kane is not the succubus, but the world behind the pages: our world.

It is one thing to recognise this demon, intellectually; to see clearly how even the purest beauty is never pure. It is another thing to actually overcome it. Typically, it is easier to blame others than to master myself. Feeling like Solomon Kane, I silence the drums and murder the succubus.

Taken as a more general ideal, what might the *ezigbo mmado* do?

The Greeks suggest a kind of competitive discipline. Plato praised the athlete Iccus of Tarentum for his equipoise: concentrating on sport so much, he was able to give up on beautiful youths. 'Such was his passion for victory, his pride in his calling, the combined fortitude and self-command of his character, that,' wrote Plato in *Laws*, 'he never once came near a woman, or a boy either, all the time he was in training.' Typical of the aristocratic Greeks, the philosopher saw *agon* — competition — as a way out of moral decadence.

In his *Symposium*, Plato also celebrated Socrates for this virtue. Socrates was known as a strong soldier, with legendary perseverance. Indeed, he once saved the life of the aristocrat Alcibiades, during the battle of Potidea — he refused to leave the wounded man, then helped him to safety. But Socrates also made morality a kind of *agon*; a sport, in which philosophical goodness was the pinnacle of athletic manhood. In *Twilight of the Idols*, Nietzsche called Socrates 'the first fencing-master' of this extreme rationality, in which becoming a chaste sage was akin to martial glory.

And this is how Socrates avoided the charms of Alcibiades, who was known for his dalliances with men and women — part of his louche party-boy persona. It seemed likely that the older, low-born, pug-faced Socrates would be desperate to screw his younger, richer, hotter student. But, no. Alcibiades tells the drinking party that he and Socrates grappled, and it came to nothing:

> I suggested we should go along to the gymna-
> sium and take a bit of exercise together, think-
> ing that something was bound to happen there.
> And would you believe it, we did our exercises
> together and wrestled with each other time and
> time again, with not a soul in sight, and still I got
> no further.

The point is not that Socrates was numbed to beauty.
He freely confesses to his 'wild-beast appetite' after seeing
the handsome Charmides, in Plato's dialogue of the same
name. This is why Nietzsche called Socrates 'a cave of every evil lust'. The point is that, with this young man and
others like Alcibiades, the Athenian mastered himself. He
turned his enormous energies inward, not outward.

Socrates was, as African philosophers might put it,
'cool'.

Promising Immensity

And if I cannot be like these Greek athletes of the soul? If
I cannot be cool in the face of beauty? Perhaps Thomas
Mann's *Death in Venice* offers a suggestion.

The German author's novel is penetrated throughout
with Platonic and Nietzschean ideas. After a professional
life of exacting precision, the novelist Gustav von
Aschenbach sees a handsome Polish youth in Venice,
and is enchanted. Like so many then and now, he is
unprepared then undone.

At first, Aschenbach tells himself that this is a
philosophical love; that Tadzio's beauty is a winged steed
to higher things. 'Eros mimicked mathematicians,' he

thinks, 'who showed dull children concrete models of abstract shapes.' From the perceivable to the intelligible — this is classic Plato.

Eventually, though, Aschenbach moves from gentle enjoyment to mania. Despite the risk of cholera in hot, wet Venice, he stays for Tadzio. And as he does, his face begins to mirror his soul. Though he earlier mocked older men for doing exactly this, Aschenbach wears cosmetics to seem younger. 'His eyes looked larger and more shiny thanks to some makeup,' Mann wrote, 'his lips that had been pale were reddened ... he beheld with excitement an ephebe in full bloom.' In other words, his physical ugliness points to another: that of his psyche, as he gives in.

By the end of the story, Aschenbach is feverish. He dreams of a Bacchanalian orgy, in which he himself is one of the mad worshippers. This is a typical Nietzschean idea, from the philosopher's first work, *The Birth of Tragedy*. For Nietzsche, the genius of tragedy was to unite two conflicting principles of life: Apolline and Dionysiac. The first is order and calm — a sober force of 'peaceful stillness'. The second, chaos and movement — all that is 'blissful ecstasy'. In his dream, Aschenbach gives in wholly to his Dionysiac urges, savouring what Mann called 'fornication and the fury of downfall'.

Eventually, Aschenbach watches Tadzio wrestling, as the handsome boy is pinned and punished for being so pretty. Then Tadzio wanders out into the sea, and turns to Aschenbach on his lounge chair:

It seemed to him the pale and lovely Summoner
out there smiled at him and beckoned; as though,
with the hand he lifted from his hip, he pointed

outward as he hovered on before into an immensity of richest expectation. And, as so often before, he rose to follow.

Both men lose their combat: Tadzio against the other boy, then Aschenbach against *eros*. Overcome by the strong arms of Dionysus, the novelist is finally vanquished — and perhaps liberated in his defeat. The 'immensity' he wades into is death.

What I am suggesting with Mann's help is this: overcoming beauty is not a job for the beautiful. They need not retreat into modesty for my sake; need not cover their 'flawless body' for fear of Solomon Kane's rapier. And they certainly need not offer themselves to me, to ease my turmoil.

Perhaps I cannot be like Socrates or the *ezigbo mmada*. Perhaps I cannot witness beauty and remain beautiful myself. If so, perhaps I ought to follow Aschenbach and just quietly die.

The Face of Nakedness

On Nudities

To begin, G was lying on her stomach, in her bra. Perhaps the bra was padded and lilac, but I cannot remember. Perhaps she was wearing black underwear. Again, I cannot remember. What I can remember is the moment she stood over me; the shock of her sudden nakedness: the long sweep from her high forehead, to high cheekbones, to high breasts.

I did not know G well. But on that afternoon she was under my dinky paper lantern, offering me her pale, leggy length; her lack of caution and sentimentality; her willingness to please, and be pleased. And emblematic of this whole afternoon — and the others that followed — was this, her nudity.

In this moment, G was novel to me. First, in the obvious sense: merely an acquaintance; someone I knew, but did not know well. Second, and more importantly: she was wholly new as this undressed, untroubled intimate, whose slight curves were foreign; whose musk was a stranger's; whose thick black hair shocked against her skin.

Unfurled from the Neck Down

I want to use hyperbole to describe this moment: 'sacred', 'holy', 'hallowed'. But these words are clumsy, lugging around the church's semantic baggage. A better word is 'spectacular', which holds on to the amazement while dropping the spiritual weight. It suggests that G's bare body was a spectacle of sorts; that those seconds, in which cotton dropped, were a special display.

(I wrote that *she* was not sentimental. I said nothing about myself.)

In his novel *The Infinities*, John Banville describes the novelty of this moment well. Old Adam is a cheater. Dying in his bed, he justifies his womanising. It was never about 'pumping away like a fireman at his hose', he says; never just the id and its organs. Instead, Adam celebrates the sorcery that transforms a public persona into private intimacy:

> How magical it was ... when the head I had
> been talking to in the street, or on a bus, or in
> the middle of a roomful of people, suddenly, in
> a shadowed bedroom, unfurled from the neck
> down this pale, glimmering extension of itself ...

Old Adam is lying, perhaps even to himself. He is rationalising his treachery, wrapping his libidinal urges in erotic and romantic paper. Still, Banville's prose is honest even if his protagonist is not: it recognises the spectacle of nakedness. What Adam remembers on his deathbed, I remember now, at my desk. Before the fucking, there was a time of baring, and this time was remarkable.

Banville also touches on why it was so remarkable. The 'extension' does not simply appear, it 'unfurls'. Similarly, G did not arrive naked. She arrived dressed, rain-drenched from the walk. Then these clothes were — smelling of deodorant and wet cotton — peeled off onto the blue carpet. Part of the 'magical' atmosphere was revelation.

But *what* was revealed? And why was it so memorable that, decades later, the scene still resonates?

To answer these questions, I want to first be clearer about what was *not* revealed: beauty, lust, sight, 'the real', or selfhood. Nakedness has such a firm grip on our psyche, I want to first loosen things a little; to do away with the obvious and the simple.

Mute Beauty

To begin, was this just my immediate response to beauty? Yes, G was beautiful — but this tells us little.

In *The Sense of Beauty*, the Spanish-born American philosopher George Santayana observed that 'beautiful' can be a confusing word. It seems to be pointing to some external fact, but it actually refers to an internal feeling. We usually distinguish deftly between our feelings and the rest of the world; we know that the tingling or throb is 'in here' while the tongue or hand is 'out there'. Beauty is the exception. We relish something, and we locate this relish in the something, not in ourselves. Santayana's definition was concise but radical: 'Beauty is pleasure regarded as the quality of a thing.'

So if beauty suggests enjoyment, what gives us joy? While scientists report some commonalities in our aesthetic ideals — symmetry as evidence of genetic health, for example — history and sociology make it clear that our pleasures are sundry. 'There is notoriously no great agreement upon aesthetic matters,' Santayana wrote, 'and such agreement as there is, is based upon similarity of origin, nature, and circumstance'. Judgements of beauty change with era and ethnicity, but also with age and state of mind. And beauty is often more an overall impression than any one mathematical ratio — we look for the gestalt, not simply this or that part. We also negotiate these gestalts: while we might have some perfect face or figure in mind, we take joy where we can find it.

So, to say that G was beautiful is to say that her sudden nakedness gave me pleasure — which is not to say much at all. It does not tell us *why* she gave me pleasure, which is far more interesting. Here, beauty is mute.

Not About Boners

Perhaps the pleasure was simple anticipation? Sex was about to happen, and my expectation draped glory over the world?

Certainly, bare skin and libido are often linked. As Ruth Barcan notes in her study *Nudity*, popular culture has a triumvirate of linked ideas: 'nakedness, sex and sin'. But are these links necessary?

A primed psyche is certainly part of the sexual mood, and this begins well before we get our kit off. The basic physiology of courtship is often about attention: singling out one human being (or two) rather than others;

highlighting their features while dimming others'. 'It puts us on alert', science journalist Joann Ellison Rodgers writes. 'It brings us the desire for desire.' During physical intimacy, alertness becomes arousal. This is a complicated psychological and biochemical process, but attention is paramount.

Testosterone, for example, does not cause an erection — it prompts men to focus on what prompts the erection. Rodgers continues: 'it's not raging hormones that arouse us initially; instead, our arousal is more likely what turns them on'. No doubt I felt this shift in consciousness with G, as she shed her bra.

But what I felt was not simply libidinal. Over the years, I have enjoyed the same feeling with other women and men — those I had no interest in screwing. It arose with J, as she wrapped herself matter-of-factly in strips of linen to pose as an odalisque; with E, as he stripped to exercise; with H, as she dropped her hospital gown. There was an eminence to these offerings of nakedness, which cannot be explained away as lust alone.

Interestingly, Homer describes a similar spectacle in the *Odyssey*. Finally safe on Phaeacia after decades at war and in exile, Odysseus bathes in a river. He is revealing, not only his body, but also his lordliness. While the water washes away his filth, the goddess Athena gives him back his physical charisma. From Alexander Pope's eighteenth century translation: 'The warrior-goddess gives his frame to shine/ With majesty enlarged, and air divine:/ Back from his brows a length of hair unfurls,/ His hyacinthine locks descend in wavy curls.' Again, the language is religious, but the point is not sectarian: there is something wonderful in the hero's nakedness, which is suddenly revealed from under filth.

The wonder of nakedness cannot be reduced to a boner.

Plural Nudities

So, when G stripped off, the revelation was neither simply her prettiness nor my horniness. Clearly, she *was* beautiful and I *was* lustful — but these are not enough to explain the moment's appeal. Something previously unseen was uncovered, but what?

I ought to be careful with this language, too. To write 'unseen' suggests that this was only visual; that the atmosphere was prompted by the sight of G's nudity — and the sight alone.

This is typical of me, and typical of European philosophy — both lean towards the visible and invisible. Our word 'theory' comes from the Greek for visual contemplation, and both Plato and Aristotle used optical metaphors for knowledge. The German-born American philosopher Hans Jonas argued that sight is especially philosophical, in that it encourages common ideas: eternity against change, essence against existence, form against matter. He ended 'The Nobility of Sight' in this way: 'the mind has gone where vision pointed'.

Alas, the mind has often gone bumblingly wrong because of this. This visual approach, what John Dewey called the 'spectator conception of knowledge', forgets our basic animality. We are not gods, watching the world from afar. We are creatures, related intimately to a vague and changing world. We do not simply look, we *experience*. And the 'true "stuff" of experience,' Dewey wrote in *Reconstruction in Philosophy*, 'is adaptive courses of action, habits, active functions, connections of doing and undergoing; sensori-motor co-ordinations.' Thinking that turns its back on this to-and-fro is thinking that falsifies our reality; that deceives with aloof simplicity.

We can discover intimacy in smell. In Angela Carter's tale 'The Tiger's Bride', a Russian girl is used by her father to pay a gambling debt. She is given to an Italian noble, a lord who hides his animality behind old-fashioned clothes, an eerie mask, and thick perfume. The Beast makes a deal: if she shows him her bare body, he will return her to her father, along with all his winnings, and more wealth. She refuses until the Beast shows his own nudity to her, then — shaking with cold and fright — she offers herself: 'I showed his grave silence my white skin, my red nipples'. But this is not the moment of most intense nakedness. This comes at the end, when the girl enters the Beast's private rooms and finds him and his simian valet without any of their typical coverings. 'There was a reek of fur and piss,' Carter writes, 'the incense pot lay broken in pieces on the floor.' This stink is far more naked for La Bestia than his actual hair. Moved by his vulnerability, the girl goes to him and offers herself in return. (He licks her with his rough tongue; licks off her many layers of civilised fakery.)

Sometimes sounds are a declaration. There was a sharp giggle of Y's, which only ever accompanied my tongue on her. This was not the levity of abandon, but kind of a wince. Y did this when pleasure became almost pain; when she was too tender or I too rough. It was like the laughter of the tickled: caught powerlessly between delight and irritation. In this, Y declared more in her voice than she did with her skin. Likewise, Ruth Barcan observes that actors nude onstage seem more naked when talking. Speech gives their bare flesh more human vulnerability.

Taste can also divulge. In Sarah Perry's novel *The Essex Serpent*, the widow Cora and a married vicar, William, consummate their affair in a forest. After her husband's abuse and the oppressions of Victorian patriarchy, Cora has long distanced herself from her physicality — and her lust. But William pulls up her skirt and kisses her belly, 'very white, marked with the silver lines her son had made'. She welcomes him, asking him to touch her — a request that seems like a ruling. William then fingers Cora, and the final revelation is as much hers as his: she is accepting, literally and figuratively, the taste of herself. 'He showed her his hand, and how she gleamed there; he put a forefinger to his mouth and hers, and they had an equal share.'

There is declaration in touch, too. Deborah Levy, in her short story 'Vienna', has a recently divorced man visiting a married woman for sex. She is 'middle Europe' to him; mysterious and luxurious and more exciting than his lonely life, missing his children. He needs his family more than he needs sex with Magret — but he still needs sex with Magret, whom he can screw but never truly be intimate with. When she strips, what surprises him is not her nudity but her temperature. 'Her long limbs are warm, he discovers, moving his cold hand between her legs and leaving it there'. For all her emotional coolness, there is a warmth to her body; a warmth that means far less than it seems to — and *this* is its meaning.

So, naked revelation — which is itself visual metaphor — is more than the seen or unseen. Nudity involves all our senses. With G, the enchantment might have equally been through my fingertips or tongue.

Draupadī

So, nakedness is more than the seen or unseen — it involves all our senses. But what exactly is sensed?

Often nakedness is confused with 'the real'; with some fundamental reality under cotton and cosmetics.

For women, especially, there is supposedly verity in the body under the clothes, the face under the make-up. As Simone de Beauvoir observed, women are expected to be nature domesticated; all the excitement of primal life, but made pretty and tame. 'He loves her rising from the sea,' she wrote in *The Second Sex*, 'and emerging from a fashionable dressmaker's establishment, naked and dressed, naked under her clothes.' And then men mock and slander women for this domestication, calling them fake; calling them liars and cheats, because they wear push-up bras or lipstick. Beneath all the artifice is reality, which men want — as long as it is youthful and safe.

In the sixteenth century, the French essayist Michel de Montaigne wrote of nudity among the New World's peoples. For him, their lack of clothes meant a lack of 'lying, treachery, dissimulation'. Putting aside the anthropological facts — often indigenous peoples were not naked at all — Montaigne's assumption is clear: dress is semblance, whereas nudity is reality. We find this metaphor throughout the history of philosophy. Nakedness was taken as proof of sin, but also of authenticity. Montaigne's contemporary in France, Jean Calvin, believed that the naked body is shameful, but necessarily so: it shows us mankind's fall from God. We need our bare genitals to witness our estrangement from the Lord. (But we also need to *not* witness this, since it encourages lust — so we wear clothes. But clothes help us forget our shame. Which encourages lust. And so on. Angst.)

The Yoruba of Western Africa have a word that captures much of this: *idí*. This is the word for 'buttocks', but also a host of other ideas, from 'reason' and 'origin' to 'secret' and 'truth'. It suggests what is normally hidden, but lies beneath. Nigerian art historian Moyo Okediji observes that *idí* is why public nudity seems proof of madness in his society: not because nakedness is rude in any straightforward sense, but because it gives too much away. To show the world your body is to lay yourself bare literally and existentially. In other words, knowledge of someone's nudity is power over them. To witness your enemy's *idí* is like knowing his arcana. 'By seeing the nakedness of his enemy,' Okediji writes in 'The Naked Truth', 'he has destroyed or reduced the potency of the enemy.'

This is one great conceit of much philosophy and patriarchal civilisation: if we can strip away all the surface layers, we get to reality beneath — especially of women. 'Femininity has often been associated,' writes Ruth Barcan, 'with triviality, passivity, inauthenticity and vanity'. In this view, under G's dress was the genuine; the actual, as opposed to the fake or artificial. To strip her was to claim The Real.

Yet the naked is no more real than the clothed, if 'real' is taken as somehow true or natural.

Think of nude dance: thoroughly artificial, a matter of talent and choreography, not some magical essence revealed. Twists and pirouettes can express with fidelity, yes. But this is because art is expressive, not because the dancers have somehow thrown away the nylon or gauze of falsehood. As Roland Barthes observed in his essay

'Striptease', the nude dancer *signifies* the natural — she does not simply offer it up, biologically. Likewise for bodybuilding physiques: they represent years of strain and often starvation, to show nerve fibres beneath usually-fatty skin. But this is neither more true than softer bodies, nor somehow more natural. It is a highly rarefied show.

Interestingly, many classical Greeks believed that their naked physiques were more civilised than clothed barbarians, because the Hellenes were *intellectually* superior. In 'Nudity in Greek Athletics', James Arieti argued that stripped runners or wrestlers were showing their mighty psyches; their power to keep their wayward cocks under control. In other words: their nakedness demonstrated cultural discipline, not some material essence.

Nudity can also be vague, rather than some clear vouchsafing. In Milan Kundera's short story 'The Hitchhiking Game', a young couple pretend to be strangers to each other: he picks her up by the side of the road, and they drive off, flirting. She pretends to be brave, and he pretends to be cruel — and each becomes this, in the bedroom. Eventually, though, she is naked. And she believes nakedness ends the pretence, because she is just herself. And she does become typically herself: shy and embarrassed. Yet her boyfriend cannot see her in this way. He only sees the girl who resists him; who refuses to be *his*. 'He didn't notice the familiar smile,' Kundera wrote, 'he saw before him only the beautiful, alien body of his own girl, whom he hated.' In this, her nudity is by no means straightforwardly true. It fools her into yielding, and him into ravaging her. This play of submission and domination is thrilling for them both, but not because she is hiding *idí* in her underpants.

This view of nakedness calls to mind a story in the *Mahābhārata*, India's foundational literary epic. Here, the princess Draupadī is 'won' in a dice game. (Yes, another woman as a prize. Misogyny is ancient and international.) Her husband Yudhiṣṭhira, after losing his brothers and himself to his enemy Duryodhana, stakes her. Angry at Draupadī's arguments, her new 'owner' asks his brother Duḥśāsana to strip Draupadī in front of her husbands and family:

> As he pulled at Draupadī's garment, another
> garment like it appeared, and this happened over
> and over again. At this, all the lords of the earth
> gave a dreadful cry as they saw this most won-
> derful sight in the world.

Nudity is like this: regardless of how many layers are pulled off, something can always be held back. Whatever was disclosed in that bedroom with G, it was not 'the real' in any simplistic sense — or no more real than her eyeliner and dress.

No Obvious Self

A similar mistake is to think nakedness reveals the self; some essential 'I' that exists below the fabric.

As David Hume observed famously in *A Treatise of Human Nature*, the self we speak of commonly is just an abstraction. We have all kinds of sensations and feelings, which seem like ours. But not one of these is *of* a self. 'I never can catch myself at any time without a perception,' Hume wrote, 'and never can observe anything but the perception'.

Importantly, his argument was not that we have no 'I' — Hume was very much himself, thankfully. His argument was that selfhood is not an object for subjects to perceive; not some thing we can stroke or bite. And if my own 'I' is no lump or bolus before me, how much more insubstantial and indistinct is someone else's? I might itemise every inch of G's flesh without ever getting closer to G herself.

In his *A Lover's Discourse*, the French philosopher and troublemaker Roland Barthes highlighted this very problem. Barthes was discussing love, not a casual fuck, but his point remains relevant here. He noted that we say someone is 'adorable' because this adorableness exists beyond all their various bits. We want to praise them in keeping with our enormous passion, and praise ourselves for this passion; for loving such a wonderful being. So we celebrate the abstraction of 'everything', which is invented behind the body. 'This *everything* he bestows upon the other in the form of a blank word,' Barthes wrote, 'for the Whole cannot be inventoried without being diminished'. A body perceived is not a self known.

Sometimes nakedness has almost nothing to do with the psyche of the naked. The *Kama Sutra* describes a woman who wants a married man, and sneakily teaches his wife lovemaking. But the bites and scratches she leaves on the wife's skin are actually 'her own signals to the man'. When the husband strips his wife he sees, not his spouse, but her rival.

The nude bodies in front of us need not say anything about themselves.

But even if I am concerned with a lover's personality, I cannot simply find it in nakedness. I might make a fetish of G's legs or wonky tooth; of her particular smirk or sighs. But these parts are nothing without the self behind them, which animates their beauty — a self that is nowhere before me.

The Face Beneath the Face

What, then, was G's nakedness? Allow me a metaphor.

In his essay on the custom of wearing clothes, Montaigne told a brief anecdote. A wealthier man asks a beggar how he wears only a shirt in winter. 'Why sir, you go with your face bare,' the beggar replies. 'I am all face.' Montaigne's sentiment involves a smug justification for poverty and privation — he was a lord, after all — but his final words are suggestive.

Naked, we are all face.

The face is not necessarily more real or true; not some obvious self; and it can be touched, tasted, smelt, heard as much as it can be seen. Perhaps the visual dominates — but never wholly. The mien is not, in short, some simple essence I can snatch and possess in a glance. I can be misled and misguided by the face; can be intrigued or inspired; can be voyeuristic or observed in turn.

Scientists like Irenäus Eibl-Eibesfeldt argue that the face has various instinctual expressions, which are also instinctually understood. In *Love and Hate*, the ethnologist noted that dilated pupils are a reflex of arousal, and hugging of a face's 'cuddliness'. Yet this does not mean the face is a straightforward truth-teller. As Eibl-Eibesfeldt himself pointed out, advertisers and demagogues alike use faces to manipulate us. And the very same instinctual expression can have various meanings: think of bared teeth in a fist fight, as against bared teeth while fucking.

Yes, the face often expresses us forcefully or subtly. It is not some public sign for private feelings — it *is* the feelings, working through our flesh. As Wittgenstein put it in his notebooks: 'The face is the soul of the body.' But, again, this does not mean the face cannot mislead or be misunderstood. (Wittgenstein himself, for all his outbursts, was frequently unintelligible to other philosophers.)

Our ideals of faces can also change. Roland Barthes once observed that Greta Garbo's face was close to a mask, whereas Audrey Hepburn's was pure personification; the former was an abstract concept, the second a specific substance. This, he wrote in 'The Face of Garbo', was 'the passage from awe to charm'. Two different faces, and two different ideas of the face itself.

This hits upon how extraordinarily expressive the face is — and how this power has little to do with some original fundament. The face is as artificial as it is natural; as deceptive as it is honest; and often more malleable than it is fixed. One mien can be even beautiful and horrific at once. Witness Marlowe's *Doctor Faustus*: Helen's face, which has Heaven in its lips, also 'launched a thousand ships/ And burnt the topless towers of Ilium'.

My point is not that nakedness *is* a face — that they are identical. The face is uniquely eloquent, and we see and seek it soon after birth. Instead, my point is that, to better comprehend nakedness, it helps to *think* of it as a face; to allow the face's character and complications to rub off on the nude.

Yet if nakedness is a face in this way, it is a second face; a new mien, which exists alongside the first. Like a friend's fraternal twin, nakedness has an exotic familiarity to it: the same, but not quite. It is often erotic, giving aesthetic pleasure. But this need not be libidinal or romantic — like a face, nakedness can delight without swollen loins or frenzied love letters.

When G stepped out of her clothes, she was introducing me to this new face: one that made her — a stranger to me — more intimate but no less foreign. Yes, this was *her* face, shot through with her unique first-person experience of the world. Yes, there was 'soul' in it, to use Wittgenstein's word. But I was not suddenly closer to this experience; not magically looking into her spirit by looking at her nude. I already recognised her face — I now recognised another, and wanted to know more.

At best, nakedness is this invitation: to learn more about the naked. This gesture is often thrilling, sure — but no less a gesture for this. It concludes nothing, finalises little but trust, provides as many questions as answers.

So, the curious joy I felt as G finally stripped: one of beginnings. The erotic equivalent of seeing a new face in a crowd.

Alone with Enki

On the Banality of Jerking Off

The black-headed man was standing in a valley. Perhaps there were waters below him; sweetwater, discoverable in caves and springs. But the soil was sandy there, and nothing grew. There were no canals, no shell middens by the shore, no herds of sheep and goats. There was not a drop of fresh water to drink. He was alone in a wasteland, listening to little but wind and his own breath.

So the man did the most obvious and helpful thing: he masturbated. '[H]e stood up full of lust like a rampant bull, lifted his penis, ejaculated and filled the Tigris with flowing water.'

So says the story of Enki in 'Enki and the World Order', told over four thousand years ago in Western Asia. The trickster-god of a freshwater lagoon, Enki made the Euphrates and Tigris rivers with his semen, and dug and filled irrigation ditches with his penis. In doing so, this divine craftsman created Mesopotamia — literally 'between rivers' in Greek — and hence civilisation itself.

To the west, during the same millennium, the Egyptians of Heliopolis believed the god Atum was similarly creative. Depending on the version of the tale, Atum either wanked the air and water gods into existence, or spat them so — having ejaculated into his own mouth.

In the *Satapatha Brahmana*, written later in Iron Age India, the great progenitor god Prajapati masturbated into Agni. Agni was his son, but also primordial fire — and the flames were hungry. There was nothing for Agni to eat. In fact, there was nothing at all, aside from Prajapati. So Prajapati made the first sacred milk, used in the Vedic sacrificial rite: the *agnihotra*. 'And Prajapati, having performed offering, reproduced himself,' reads Julius Eggeling's Victorian translation, 'and saved himself from Agni, Death, as he was about to devour him.'

So, the world here begins sophomorically: with a dude tugging himself, and offering his cum to the world like a birthday present.

I told Ruth about this, Enki's gift: 'How like a man,' she said with a half-smile.

Touching Nothing

Compare this to the biblical cosmogony: the Lord simply speaks. There is clay later, of course; and Eve, formed from a rib. But before anything, there is a sky sprite who is more sigh than flesh: 'The Spirit of God moved upon the face of the waters.' The god does not travel on foot. His *ruach* or spirit — from the Hebrew for 'breath' — soars. So this deity is no craftsman, shaping the cosmos with his calloused fingers. And he is certainly no wanker, spilling cum to help make the earth fertile. The heir to Near Eastern animist beliefs, the Lord is one of atmospheres; one whose power is like winds. His speech makes things so. 'God said, Let the earth bring forth grass, the herb yielding seed, and the fruit tree yielding fruit after his kind, whose seed is in itself, upon the earth,' reads *Genesis*. 'And it was so.'

So Hebrew and Christian myth begins as the very antithesis of Enki and his fellow jerk-offs: the Holy Spirit is a hands-off creator.

There are countless other creation myths, of course. Eggs are popular. A first man in Chinese myth, Pangu, is born of a cosmic egg. The Egyptian god Khnum creates another such egg on his potter's wheel. In Tibet, the divine egg's shell becomes cliffs, and the yolk a life-filled lake. Many stories also feature divers, plucking primordial stuff from below. In Indigenous North American, Central Asian and Hindu myths, a beast swims into the primal ocean and brings up the earth. Two more metaphors: bodies torn apart, and bodies coming together. In Scandinavian poetry, a primordial being is ripped to bits. 'Out of Ymir's flesh was fashioned the earth,/ And the mountains were made of his bones,' the giant Vafthruthnir tells Odin. And in Hesiod's *Theogony* — which also features dismemberment — Eros exists from the get-go, and sex begins as soon as there are divinities to enjoy it. '[O]f Night were born Aether and Day,' Hesiod wrote, 'whom she conceived and bare from union in love with Erebus.' These do not feature masturbation, but they are certainly fleshy: their gods break, swim, tear, screw, and so on.

There is magical speech elsewhere. The Memphis god Ptah — also a patron of craftsmen — talks the nine great divinities into existence. '[E]very word of the god came into being,' says the Shabaka Stone, 'through the thoughts in the heart & the command by the tongue.' But note the metaphors: this god has a mouth to speak, and blood to be pumped. And this story was told alongside many other tales of fucking, killing, and — once again — wanking. The god Min-Horus was praised at coronation ceremonies, when the king had to ejaculate for good luck. 'The king was supposed to literally produce the seed of life,' David Leeming writes, 'which would ensure the annual flooding of the Nile.'

For me, the contrast between Enki and Jehovah is stunning. Of all the ways to begin a world, these are diametrically opposed. The Lord suggests aloof ethereality: no soiled palms, no semen. Enki touches himself, whereas the Holy Spirit barely touches anything.

A Rare Hobby

Each of these stories is part of an enormous mythic world, rich with symbolism. Myth, Roberto Calasso says, 'is always a tree with many branches'. The twig that most intrigues me here is this: the tales of Enki, Atum, and Prajapati celebrate jerking off. Masturbation is neither private nor vilified; neither something to hide nor regret. Instead, it becomes something to praise. Not because it is moral or beautiful, but because it is a glorious work of creation.

This contrasts with the story of Genesis, in which the world begins with breath and words, not tugging and cum. For the Hebrews, all matter was dross until it was animated and consecrated by divine winds. And this outlook only grew more fervent in later Christian thought and practice: our very animality or physicality was suspect. For Christians, as Nietzsche put it: 'body is despised and hygiene is denounced as sensual; the church even ranges itself against cleanliness'. Here, sexuality became another devilish and dangerous part of the flesh. While Jews tended to see screwing as a healthy part of life, the followers of Christ were more wary. There was a 'tension between salvation and pleasure,' as historian James Brundage put it, 'a gloomy suspicion that the one cannot be attained without renouncing the other.' Desire was especially troubling. Procreative intercourse was *allowable*, but lust was simply bad. For church fathers like Ambrose, Jerome, and Augustine, you may fuck out of duty — but you may not fuck with delight. (Jerome: 'It is disgraceful to love another man's wife at all, or one's own too much.') As classicist Kathy Gaca puts it in *The Making of Fornication*, 'sexual pleasure within and outside of Christian marriage is the darkness of evil, death, and damnation'. In this outlook, masturbation was most certainly a sin. Yes, it was tolerated as a lesser evil — but it was an evil nonetheless.

And it was almost never treated as something good and great, as it was in Enki's tale; something worthy of civilised creation.

Faced with the body-denying Christian legacy, I also want to praise wanking. Like many moderns, I see it as normal and healthy. And this is not just wishful thinking: turning a lazy pull into therapy. Current research reveals that regular masturbation is good for us, physiologically and psychologically. A review of studies by physiologist Roy Levin reported that jerking off can, among other things, bolster men's immune systems, ease women's period pain, and slow genital atrophy. In fact, masturbation might also encourage what human sexuality professor Eli Coleman calls 'ownership, control and autonomy' over our own bodies, *and* help us enjoy better intimacy with our loved ones. At the absolute least, wanking is that truly rare hobby: a cheap, harmless thrill.

Perhaps mischievously, I also want to stifle others' pleasure. Not the wankers — let them revel in themselves. No, I want to ruin the joy of any remaining priggish sermonisers, who are cursing or controlling masturbation. As French philosopher Michel Foucault noted in an interview, there is 'enjoyment in intervening' — an enjoyment religious leaders and parents have indulged for centuries. They have savoured their power over others' bodies.

May this perverse thrill die.

Libidinous Massage

Before I hurl myself heroically to its defence, I ought to define what I mean by 'masturbation'.

I am not discussing masturbating others, or with others. Even if the techniques are exactly the same, the practice is not. Witness Leopold Bloom in James Joyce's *Ulysses*, pulling himself at the beach while watching Gerty MacDowell. The moment Gerty meets Leopold's gaze, then shows him her legs and underwear, a relationship exists that is more than voyeurism; more than the tiny consciousness of one man and his fantasy. 'She let him,' Joyce writes, 'and she saw that he saw'. To jerk off a lover, or with a lover, is to encounter another human being, intimately. It can be fully romantic. So, the solitary wanker is doing something very different from the couple or threesome. And it is the solitary wanker — Enki, creating Mesopotamia with his ejaculate — that interests me here.

And what exactly is masturbation? Dictionary definitions and etymologies are little help. In English, 'masturbation' first pops up in a 1603 translation of Montaigne's essays, and refers (uncoincidentally) to a philosopher: 'Diogenes in sight of all, exercising his Maisterbation'. While its origins are dim, 'masturbate' comes from Latin, perhaps from *manus* (hand) and *stuprare* (to defile).

Leaving aside the idea of defilement for now, the *manus* part is misleading. While hands and fingers are our most common ways of pleasuring ourselves, we can also get off with pillows, teddy bears, spa jets, saddles, or simply with the thighs. This is to say nothing of the various things used in the hands — from the more obvious vibrators and mechanical vaginas, to the more *outré* Issey Miyake perfume bottles, Ken dolls, pork loins, hammers. The *Kama Sutra* recommends 'a squash, a lotus stalk, or a bamboo section' alongside dildos of metal and wood. From *Portnoy's Complaint*: '"Come, Big Boy, come," screamed the maddened piece of liver that … I bought one afternoon at a butcher shop and … violated behind a billboard.' When we masturbate, we stimulate ourselves sexually — whether we do this with fingertips, carpentry tools, or figurines is neither here nor there. For the same reason, slang is also little help: tugging, flicking the bean, jerking, rubbing one out, pulling, low fiving, all chiefly refer to hand movements. 'Onanism' is named for the biblical man who ejaculated on the ground, instead of in his sister-in-law, Tamar. But this is *coitus interruptus*, not masturbation.

Masturbation need not involve fantasy, but these are often mistakenly paired. Indeed, for Enlightenment philosopher Immanuel Kant, illusion was one of the onanist's many vices. In his *Doctrine of Virtue,* Kant argued that jerking off is 'unnatural' because we get horny over fake objects instead of real ones. And in this way, we 'bring forth a desire contrary to nature's end'. Put simply, masturbation ends in orgasm but not procreation, because the beloved is mental not physical. And this is against the order of things, because our genitals are made — note the assumption — to have babies in wedlock.

Kant's very Christian notion is false because it gets biology profoundly wrong — we are not 'made' for anything, and daydreaming and conception are not automatically at odds. (*In vitro* fertilisation actually requires Maisterbation.) Kant is also wrong because he assumes we must jerk off with the help of lusty mirages, which take us away from our intimates.

Yes, we often fantasise, and men more so than women. But we can also picture our lovers, instead of forbidden others or random strangers. And we need not picture anyone at all: in the right mood, friction is enough for many. Asexuals commonly wank for what researchers call 'physical needs' — they are horny for touch, but not for the touch of another person.

What of those who orgasm from fantasy alone? Is not this illusion *as* masturbation? In short, no. This is simply the waking equivalent of a wet dream. We can climax without wanking, or wank without climax — the little death is proof of nothing here.

So, masturbation need not involve hands, fantasy, or orgasm. At its simplest, it is the sexual stimulation of ourselves. And it is 'sexual' because the pleasure is more than just muscular or epidermic. It involves the physiology of arousal. Yes, masturbation can also be romantic or erotic; can involve intimacy with another human being, or a receptivity to beauty. But it need not.

In essence, jerking off is libidinous massage of oneself.

Nothing to Be Ashamed of

So, masturbation is just ordinary rubbing — with arousal. What is wrong with this?

I have already dealt with some of Kant's problems with wanking: that it involves fantasy, and that this distracts us from our 'natural' ends. Both are false.

Another charge is vulgarity, though this was made against all pagan sexuality, rather than just jerking off. Clement of Alexandria mocked the licentiousness and violence of the Greek divinities, for example. 'The father of gods and men, according to you,' he wrote in his second-century *Exhortation to the Heathen*, 'was so given to sexual pleasure, as to lust after all, and indulge his lust on all, like the goats of the Thmuitæ.' Clement also lambasted the Greek worship of statues ('dead matter shaped by the craftsman's hand'), as against the purely mental sight of God. The Alexandrian's outlook was typically ethereal, seeing sin in the pagans' surrender to the flesh.

But Clement and his brethren were wrong, as Christian scripture — to say nothing of Christian history — is full of barbarity and lust. The Hebrew bible is bloody with massacres, violations, tortures. Christ's own death is a brutal agony. And to this day, Catholics eat and drink their lord, symbolically. My point is not that Christians are louche cannibals, but that their myths are still myths — and crudity is a large part of the mythic consciousness. The coarse and the refined often come together in origin tales, alongside the holy and profane, raw and cooked, wild and domestic, and so on. The Christian God is, as historian Mircea Eliade put it in *Myths, Rites, Symbols*, 'terrible and gentle at once' — and his sanctity *is* this unity. Trickster-gods like Enki and Christ create by transgressing; they cross boundaries, literally and figuratively. In other words, it is no surprise to find crudeness in myth, and masturbation is no more or less vulgar than the Christian holy books.

Another argument against masturbation is that wanking is somehow 'against nature'; that it breaks some cosmic law. But this is false in any interpretation. Many other species get themselves off. Stallions flex their stomach muscles, bouncing their cocks against their guts. Some orang-utans rub their clitorises with sticks, and porcupines their cloacas with pinecones. Turtles get their rocks off against stones. So, if by 'natural' we mean 'nonhuman', then masturbation is thoroughly natural. If 'God made the wild animals of the earth of every kind, and the cattle of every kind, and everything that creeps upon the ground of every kind,' he also made them horny.

If by 'natural' we only mean some special 'human nature', then this is also dodgy. Kant argued that rubbing ourselves made us 'below the level of beasts', sullying our rational liberty with bestial urges. Yet the philosopher gave no reasons why masturbation did this, but not other everyday customs. He was fine with supping on beef, sipping on coffee and wine, puffing on tobacco — in moderation, of course. Why not jerking off in moderation? He was also fine with manual labour, in which workers, he said, toiled without losing themselves. If I can use my body for a boss's profit, surely I can use my own body as an 'instrument for … satisfaction'? Kant's criticisms of masturbation were less about ethics and more about eighteenth-century bourgeois fear of idleness and fragile masculinity.

One final criticism of wanking is that it is self-directed rather than other-directed; that it turns us away from other human beings or God. It sends the man 'back into the prison of himself,' wrote Christian author CS Lewis in a letter, 'there to keep a harem of imaginary brides'. Again, fantasy and jerking off are not the same thing, and fantasy can be enjoyed for its own sake — we enjoy the illusion, then return to the world.

But more importantly, Lewis's 'prison' would be a problem if sex were only for communication with others, or communion with divinities or nature. But sex is no one thing: it can be everything from simple instinctual urge to full existential encounter, and these values are not mutually exclusive. We can easily enjoy tender lovemaking in the morning, then a quick pull in the evening, and the only commonality is libido. There is no conflict, no contradiction. As Alan Soble puts it in his essay 'Masturbation, Again,' 'sexual desire is the desire for certain pleasurable sensations, period.' That we satisfy this desire with a few movements of the hand, pillow, or scent bottle is no proof of egotism or narcissism.

In short: masturbation is neither especially vulgar (when compared to the holy scriptures), nor unnatural, nor selfish. While Christian myth prevailed over the millennia, the story of Enki was closer to the truth: wanking is nothing to be ashamed of.

Magnificent Gift, Ugly Curse

As in the myth of Enki, many moderns now celebrate masturbation. We might find it laughable or embarrassing; we might prefer it to happen privately and quietly. But this ubiquitous pastime is no longer seen as vicious or evil; not that hideous vice by which a man 'sets aside his person and degrades himself below the level of animals', as Kant lectured. While it hardly needs repeating (given my prose style), I share this commitment to jerking off.

And yet. I am not wholly comfortable with the Mesopotamian vision of masturbation. Not because it is archaic or lewd, but because it is still oddly conservative. When it comes to wanking, Egyptian myth and Christian ethics are closer than they might seem.

To begin, they are both patriarchal. In fact, most of the cosmogonies share a commitment to male domination. The great creator is usually a dude, establishing a masculine universe with his power or flesh. Bards or scribes are born of women, but the mythic worlds they sing or write of — and the laws and customs they justify — are typically born of men. And in those tales where feminine gods or principles rule, these are often overthrown. More misogynist fiction than historical fact, the ancient matriarchy exists chiefly to be usurped. 'Men have shaped for their own exultation great virile figures,' Simone de Beauvoir writes, '... woman has only a secondary part to play in the destiny of these heroes.' This is certainly true of Enki, whose daughters chiefly exist to make more daughters. If these men are beaten, it is usually by other men — the basic logic remains. Enki's paganism and the Lord's Christianity are patriarchal bedfellows.

More subtly, both stories see masturbation as enormously powerful. Yes, they conflict over the value of this might: Mesopotamia in favour, the church against. And behind this conflict is another, which is metaphysical. As a Sumerian water spirit, Enki is fluid and fertile; he gushes and seeps and spurts. He is the emblem of a culture in which, as classicist Keith Dickson writes, 'irrigation and intercourse [are] interchangeable tropes'. As a Platonic sky spirit, the Christian Lord is ethereal; he soars and hovers from afar. He symbolises the promise of a perfect universe, while our world jets and spills. Here, 'the earthly world is condemned to eternal decay', as philosopher Arran Gare puts it, describing Augustine's City of God. In masturbation, these tendencies come to a head: one for all that is pulsing and squirting, another for all that is untainted and unmoving. Yet despite this strife, these mythic visions both treat wanking as a primal force, which achieves vast things when liberated. It can build the foundations of civilisation; it can demolish them. It is generative, physically; it is degenerative, spiritually. It is a magnificent gift; it is an ugly curse.

All this, just from wanking. An enormous potential is suggested, awaiting realisation in each of us — with just a few rubs.

Diogenes' Face

I confess, my immediate response to the myths of Enki, Atum and Prajapati was: really? Of all the ways to make the world or its divinities, *this*? We look back aeons, before inscriptions on stone; before the memories of the aged; before there were even human beings, in an era of hazy, fleeting dreams — and we find wanking? Masturbation seems so at odds with this antediluvian atmosphere of magic and superhuman will.

Yes, I welcome the Mesopotamian, Egyptian and Vedic celebration of masturbation; their willingness to depict this pastime without cringe or flinch. They give the gods a very human habit. But they also give these gods too much kudos for this habit. This is better than Christian primness, to be sure — but still farcical to me, because it shares with orthodox Christianity a mistaken belief in the potency of jerking off.

In fact, what distinguishes wanking is its simplicity and ease.

All of the mythic origins other than masturbation are *achievements*. Even if we are blasé libertines, coupling with another being is a notable event. Likewise for all the other mythic beginnings: violence, great cosmic eggs, diving deep. These are all accomplishments of sorts, which ask for some striving — if only psychologically. They ask us to exist, however briefly, beyond ourselves.

By contrast, wanking is unexceptional and unchallenging for most of us. With or without climax, it is not a notable event. Because it is merely libidinal massage, it involves almost no physical or mental labour. Hence Diogenes' famous quip: 'When behaving indecently in the marketplace, he wished it were as easy to relieve hunger by rubbing an empty stomach.' The philosopher scandalised the public by doing a private thing publicly, but the thing itself was banal: a few minutes' work, for simple satisfaction. As jerk-offs, we know precisely what we are doing: *this* rhythm; *that* gentleness or roughness; *those* daydreams, *these* fictional selves. Poet Jessica McKenna, in 'Ease of Use': 'It's a quick thing –/ Five or so all rubbed out/ In five minutes or less.' Yes, we can tease ourselves; can punctuate and prolong the joy — but these are exactly the pauses we want.

Perhaps this is not true for some teenagers or older naïfs, first fumbling with their own bits. Witness teenager Holly in Ibi Kaslik's novel *Skinny*: 'Hey. It's a little button, a tiny electric button.'

And even for more experienced adults, physical transformations can make masturbation baffling. Samantha Allen, writing for *Splinter* magazine: 'Having to navigate a vagina was like being plucked out of preschool and placed in a quantum physics course overnight.' While Allen knew exactly what to do with a penis, her new post-operative bits were a mystery. Likewise for journalist Ana Valens, who tried jerking off after hormone replacement therapy. 'It's like I can't figure out how this thing works,' she wrote in *Daily Dot*.

Masturbation can also feel enormously liberating for those raised with conservative guilt; for those taught that their pleasures turned their faces from God's loving gaze. This is especially so for women, whose wanking was doubly sinful: as purely for pleasure, and as female pleasure *at all*. While classical and Medieval medical texts recommended rubbing the clitoris to relieve pent-up fluids (their 'semen'), theologians were typically less generous. Witness the influential Anglo-Saxon penitential of Theodore, which recommended three years' penance for jilling off. Even when never said aloud, the Christian commands against sexual discovery are aggressive, and they continued well into the modern era. Consider Eleanor in Adam Roberts's *Swiftly*. For all her education and curiosity, this nineteenth-century Briton is wary of pleasuring herself. 'She felt a disinclination to touch herself between her thighs, as if it were somehow wrong or shameful,' Roberts writes, 'and yet she could not remember ever having been specifically rebuked for doing so.' Generations later, in America's south, the silent prohibition remains. 'I feel like us been doing something wrong,' says Alice Walker's Celie in *The Color Purple*, after rubbing herself alongside Shug.

But for those of us with decades of guiltless practice under our belts, masturbation is neither challenge nor chore. It is banal. It is worth doing, and worth enjoying — but not worth praising as an epic deed, or fearing as a cosmic vice. And more importantly, this is fine. After many centuries of ethical and metaphysical damnation; after charges of corruption and sin; after shame and even criminalisation — after, in short, wearing a grand satanic persona, masturbation takes off the mask to reveal: Diogenes' calm face.

Putting Aside Grandiosity

My feelings about masturbation are ambiguous, and an analogy with reading AJ Ayer might help. (Yes, I did just write those words.)

Alfred 'Freddie' Jules Ayer was an English philosopher, whose youthful work *Language, Truth, and Logic* scandalised philosophy in the years between the world wars. This slim book popularised in English the ideas of logical positivism, a school of thought developed a decade earlier — chiefly in Germany and Austria. The manifesto shocked thinkers, not so much for what it included, but for what it excluded: much of philosophy.

The gist of Ayer's argument was straightforward: meaningful statements come in two kinds, analytic and synthetic. The first include mathematics and logic, the second worldly facts. The first ask for proofs, the second for evidence. 'We say that a sentence is factually significant to any given person, if, and only if,' he wrote, 'he knows how to verify the proposition which it purports to express.'

Ayer's point, made with excitement and charm, was that many philosophical statements cannot be verified. They *seem* to be talking about the world, but what they discuss can neither be proven nor evidenced. Put another way, the problem with most intellectual endeavours is not that they are false, but that they cannot even be falsified. In fact, Ayer said, many of the great scholarly works were simply meaningless: nonsense texts, which left us more fantasists than philosophers. These intellectuals were right to think, but their thinking got away with them. Their speculations — learned and highly technical — turned into fancies. Witness Ayer on god (any popular deity will do):

> to say that 'God exists' is to make a metaphysical utterance which cannot be either true or false. And by the same criterion, no sentence which purports to describe the nature of a transcendent god can possess any literal significance.

Goodbye, millennia of theology.

As it happens, logical positivism was also gone within a few decades — Ayer himself noted the shortcomings of his 'young man's book'. The most obvious problem was that its basic concepts were, by its own definition, 'meaningless' — neither analytic nor synthetic. How can you verify the principle of verifiability? It also ignored the enormous human context needed to make sense of any human statement; the 'ways of life' later made famous by Wittgenstein, an early fellow traveller of Ayer.

Still, I find the mood of *Language, Truth, and Logic* emancipating. It looks over the centuries, takes a deep breath (probably of a cigarette, from a silver case) and says: 'nah'. It does not just take issue with this or that argument; with a concept here or fact there. It concludes that many of the most legendary arguments in history were, at bottom, absurd. All that anxiety, rancour, regret; all the name-calling and politicking; all the reputations balancing delicately upon a treatise or sermon — all about nothing. Despite the author's confessed 'passion', there is a calmness to Ayer's manifesto; a sense that I no longer need to be sitting on the edge of my seat, worrying about Plato's Forms, Hegel's Absolute, Heidegger's Being.

I am no follower of Freddie's. But I am drawn to this sweeping gesture, which disposes of angst and condemnation; which clears away so many years of needless concern. I want to do for masturbation what he did for philosophy and theology: ease the tension. A similar calm ought to settle upon jerking off. As with the grand history of ideas, I recognise the worth of masturbation, and have no wish to see it made a monster or villain. I have a fondness for it, in much the same way that I have a fondness for Neoplatonism or the Christian mysticism. But this is a fondness for something that, after so many centuries, can finally be seen as ordinary. This is emancipation through the quotidian: masturbation is good but banal. It is more hobby or therapy than cosmic rite.

As a modern, it is oddly liberating to finally put aside all the grandiosity; to turn epochal cosmogony or sin into a humble daily deed; to raise the sluice gates, and allow the mythic and religious waters to ebb away. I need neither their Christian vapours nor their Mesopotamian floods.

I showed Ruth these final lines, on the simple banality of masturbation. She replied, smiling again: 'How like a man.'

Fuckzilla

On Necessity, Freedom and Huge Robot Penises

She is alone in an industrial room. Exposed metallic surfaces, functional lights built into the steps, large numbers on the wall in digital sans-serif font. She is wearing a teal crop top, white skirt, black pumps with enormous heels. Her hair is brushed-on blonde, straight, recently styled. She has tattoos: massed blooming roses, an owl, a welding torch, a raven and skull, a cupcake.

Why is she here?

She toys with her skirt's hem. Bites her finger and lip, then widens her eyes. She is looking up coyly, but smiling knowingly. These are all what Eibl-Eibesfeldt called 'typical elements of human flirting behavior'. From Japan to Germany, Papua to New York, they are quickly comprehended signs of courtship. They demonstrate not only availability, but also interest: *I am aroused by you*.

So, she is here for sex. Or, rather: for the pornographic fantasy of sex.

Sure enough, the script plays out with typical swiftness: from teasing to masturbation. The actress sits on a stool, spreads her legs wide, and begins rubbing herself with a large, loud vibrator. Grinning. Sighing. Moaning. Hunching over, laughing.

Next, as always: penetration. On all fours atop a padded metal cage, she is screwed doggy style. The actress moans, cries, points her toes. She sounds almost pained; as if the stimulation were too much. *Almost*. Yet there is no ambiguity in this fantasy: as the thing plunges in and out of her, she is given over to her own pleasure.

But there is no cock. Within the narrative at least, there are no other human beings in that industrial room. The phallus is actually a thick pink dildo on a long metal crankshaft, driven by an electric motor. It slows down and speeds up throughout the video, but it never stops.

There is no climactic cumshot; no scenes of the actress doting on frenulum or testicles; no whispered or grunted words. She is being fucked by a machine named Intruder — what the video advertises as the 'best fuck of her life'.

Unmoved, Untroubled

While I am watching Intruder do its job, various thoughts arise.

I think about how many hours the actress has invested in her tattoos. In his *Pensées*, Pascal noted: 'the sole cause of man's unhappiness is that he does not know how to stay quietly in his room.' This pornographic actress is a Pascalian exemplar. She knows how to sit quietly in a room.

I think about the model's abdominal strength, as she holds herself up for the camera. Private sex usually involves lots of physical negotiation, as lovers seek pleasure without distracting aches or cramps. This actress is paid to keep herself stimulated but always available. From her vulva and anus, to the stretch marks and fine down on her arse, she is in high definition display — not because she needs to be, but because the viewer supposedly needs her to be. This is what cinema scholar Linda Williams, in *Hard Core*, calls the 'meat shot': proof that real genitals are involved, and they are really swollen and wet.

I think about the cast and crew. Did the actress do her own hair and make-up? How many staff are hired to design, build, and clean the set? Do they have an electrician or engineer on call, in case the motor blows or camshaft cracks? A doctor or paramedic, in case of injury? I hope the studio is full of professionals, whose labour is valued by one another if not by polite company. (Bourgeois talents, *demi-monde* jobs.)

I offer these thoughts, not because they are especially noteworthy, but because their mere existence is. A model is naked and writhing in front of me, and I am thinking about a French mathematician, exercise, and professional status. More curiously: I am thinking *at all*.

As Georges Bataille notes in *Eroticism*, arousal is not a workaday mood. Being horny messes up my vocational world of neat plans and schedules; it forsakes 'lucid and distinct awareness' for a lurching, throbbing mind. But viewing this video, I am basically at work. My psyche is unmoved, untroubled. Not a single pulse of arousal gets between me and my thoughts.

Perhaps I am physically into this, but just mentally distracted? Research reveals that pornography viewers can certainly show the signs of titillation — greater blood flow to the genitals — without feeling so. As so often happens in sexuality, there can be a break between subjective psychology and objective chemistry; a sense that the flesh wants what the mind avoids. But this occurs far more often with women than with men. In their meta-analysis for *Archives of Sexual Behaviour*, Meredith Chivers and colleagues reported that men are consistently more aware of their boners. (Understatement of the millennium.)

Yet even if I were more tumescent than I knew, this would not change my mind. As I watch the actress getting what the video claims is the 'best fuck of her life', I do not want to get off — I simply want to comprehend.

Part of this comprehension is the realisation that, to others, I am as empty as this pornographic scene. However amorous my consciousness is to myself, I am a sexual void to many. My point is not that they find me creepy or gross — although some no doubt have, or do. (In high school, I used explicit rap lyrics to make myself seem mature. In doing so, I failed.) My point is that seeing another being as sexual is psychological work, and not everyone invites this labour.

With this model and her Intruder, however, it is a good opportunity: to reflect, without lust getting in the way.

Two Modes

What is there to comprehend about the Intruder? For many viewers, the advertised fantasy is seemingly enough. They believe that this is indeed the 'best fuck', and they can enjoy the spectacle. Commenters on the video say 'I better go and get a robotic dick then', 'the male species is obsolete', and 'she no longer wants a human man'. In short: the Intruder is understood as pleasure, pure and simple.

But for me, this spectacle is more complicated. To begin, it is not simply masturbation. While the film includes the actress rubbing herself with underwear, a finger, or vibrator, this is only the beginning; the foreplay before consummation. After she touches herself, the actress is touched. In other words, the supposed highlight of the video is something *being done to her*.

My point is not that she is merely a thing of misogynistic fantasy, what feminist John Stoltenberg calls a 'mindless fuck tube' in 'How Men Have (a) Sex'. My point is that this scene involves two quite different modes of sex: masturbation of oneself, then masturbation by another. The first mode is an eroticised solitude, where the actress's performed pleasure — real or simulated — invites the audience's. Perhaps she is directed to stroke thus or whimper thus, but the scene is simple enough: one model and her jollies.

The second mode suggests a relationship between fucked and fucker; a dynamic, which involves more than a lone model and her toy.

If the model has a relationship of sorts with these things, what exactly is this a relationship with?

Robots

Many see these devices as 'sex robots'. This is a clumsy use of the word, but helpful in other ways.

Strictly speaking, only machines with some autonomy are robots. They are designed and often manufactured by human beings, but they sense, analyse, and move on their own.

Because of our anthropocentric bent, we often have trouble seeing the autonomy in these alien things. A vibrator might look like a rounded bottle opener, but be a genuine robot: with pressure, movement and heat sensors, and a computer which changes its rhythms with our arousal. In contrast, fake eyes and a rubber cock on motorised tracks might look humanoid. But if this machine is controlled remotely by some dude, it is just another gadget. Anthropomorphic machines, with their suggestion of sentience, invite ideas of futuristic android coupling. But they are merely props, lacking even autonomy, let alone actual artificial intelligence.

What these fuck machines have in common with robots is necessity. Necessity is what *must* happen — the stuff of basic physics and biology. It cannot be negotiated with or threatened to stop. It cannot be glibly cajoled. We *must* breathe oxygen and exhale carbon dioxide; *must* eat and drink and excrete; *must* age and die; *must*, in most cases, rot away. And well before the end, most of us feel that we *must* have sex, if not babies. Necessity is the ceaseless urgency of existence, what Hannah Arendt called, in *The Human Condition*, the 'gigantic circle of nature ... where all natural things swing in changeless ... repetition.' The ancient Greek goddess of necessity was named Ananke. As Calasso observes, she had very few temples: why pray to a deity who will never listen?

Necessity just does what she does, oblivious to pleas and commands alike.

And how did the Greeks work with Ananke; with the drudgery of filthy homes, carpentry workshops, copper mines? Slaves. While free men — and they were *only* men — steered the great ship of state, thralls were scrubbing the deck and bailing out seawater. 'Because men were dominated by the necessities of life,' Arendt continued, 'they could win their freedom only through the domination of those whom they subjected to necessity by force.' This was so ordinary, Aristotle believed that many were 'slaves by nature', as he put it in his *Politics*. Lacking thought and speech, they existed to be ruled. The thralls were not rational animals — they were 'living tools'.

Aristotle also wondered about tools that *seemed* alive: technological slaves, with no souls. 'If every instrument could accomplish its own work, obeying or anticipating the will of others,' he wrote, 'chief workmen would not want servants, nor masters slaves.' In Aristotle's Athens, these only existed in fiction. In Homer's *Iliad*, Hephæstos the god of metallurgy wrought tripods that walked on their own: 'self-moved, obedient to the beck of gods'.

Today, we have these mythical instruments as part of everyday life. They can wash our dirty sheets, vacuum up our skin cells. And they can cause the orgasms that soil our linen and chafe our groins. They buzz, pump and suck, hopefully prompting what science journalist Joann Ellison Rodgers calls 'a firestorm of immensely rewarding, blissful physiological and psychological events, fueled by neurotransmitters and hormones.' Much of this activity is opaque to us, working without our choice or even knowledge. But if we are in the mood, it works — and often stubbornly, even savagely. This much heat and pressure; these angles and those rhythms, and our flesh responds automatically. So, by controlling the necessities of electromagnetism and chemistry, we bring on necessities within ourselves. We make something that *must* happen

— or at least that feels this way, once it is underway.

In other words, we now have Hephæstos's fictional instruments at our beck. And our popular word for these is surprisingly apt: robots. In his play *R.U.R.*, Czech author Karel Čapek called his artificial servants *robota*, from the Slavic word for forced labour. If fuck machines are indeed 'robots', it is because they continue this ancient legacy of control: human beings, making other beings deal with necessity. Obviously there is an enormous ethical difference between captive people and engineered things, but both are answers to the same fundamental question. Whether these beings are biological or mechanical, for cleaning or climaxing, the basic idea is the same: they labour with Ananke, so we need not.

The Face of What Must Be

So, the Intruder and its comrades are not exactly robots — but they exemplify robotic logic. They are engines of necessity, with a special difference: they are supposed to evoke necessities in us. And these necessities are sharable. If all goes well, the fuck machine encourages arousal in the model, whose pleasure encourages arousal in the viewer, whose arousal encourages arousal in her lover, and so on. Horniness can be daisy-chained. (Though not to this philosopher.)

Yet there is more to this pornography than simple pleasure. It is not simply *that* the actress is wet and moaning, but *how*. For this spectacle, it matters that the penetrator or vibrator is a machine.

What the fuck machine offers here is indeed a relationship, and a strange one: a spectacle of coupling without a couple. In reality, this is masturbation. With help from the crew, the actress is using these machines — just as she might use a hair dryer before the shoot. But in cinematic fantasy, this is a robot screwing a model.

Alongside the Intruder, these machines have names like Assblaster, Monster, and The Little Guy — all suggesting personality. Perhaps the most evocative is Fuckzilla, which looks like a cliché science fiction robot: glowing, telescopic eyes over caterpillar tracks, a long dildo arm and a chainsaw of synthetic tongues. These beings have no psyche, no self, no character. But they suggest a personality with their macho names, and performances in the videos: unfeeling, unstoppable, yet somehow uncannily causing orgasms.

In this way, the fuck machine *personifies what must be*. Its inner life — which exists purely in fiction — is filled to brimming with necessity.

Prometheus Unbound

Just how necessary is necessity? As it happens, history is a story of Ananke's gradual flight from her throne. Not because we have somehow done away with necessity, but because her kingdom has shrunk.

For the ancient Greeks, Necessity was absolutely sovereign; the great dread goddess, holding her spindle of fate. The sixth-century poet Simonides wrote: 'The gods themselves strive not against *ananke*.' His point was not that deities were respectful citizens, but simply that they were not omnipotent — for all their power, they were not strong enough to overcome destiny. Even Zeus, mighty father of the gods, bowed to this divinity: 'He cannot fly from Fate,' said Prometheus in Aeschylus' *Prometheus Bound*.

In the centuries since, for good or ill, we have gained greater mastery over the physical world. The 'laws' of physics, chemistry, and biology have been described in precise detail, and much of the planet can be controlled and usually predicted. We also have a greater idea of the 'laws' of psyche and society, understood as regular tendencies not absolute rules.

In this modern vision of the universe, necessity is no longer fate: we can follow causes and effects to their conclusions — however complex — but we no longer believe these conclusions *had to be* all along; that there is a plan, blueprint or charter for existence.

Take orgasm. It can feel fated; like it absolutely must and will happen. Think of Nan in Sarah Waters' *Tipping the Velvet*, coming as Florence fists her: 'I think I called out — I think I shivered and panted and called out.' Observe the 'I think': Nan is not wholly in control of her own movements — or even aware of them. So much of this is automatic: contractions in the genitals, the release of hormones, neurotransmitters and enzymes in the brain and groin. There are rhythms in climax, and rhythms in our interest: from the spasms in our muscles (just less than a second between each), to the monthly cycles that leave us more or less horny. These are all forms of necessity, in that they are instinctual and physically determined.

But suppose we are drunk? Or our child cries? Or we are simply tired, and suddenly anxious about work? An orgasm can always cease to be, along with our whole erotic mood. It is also possible to cum without a buzz, or to have the psychological euphoria without the contractions. What we think of as a typical climax is a complicated balance of stimulation, chemistry, and state of mind — and a change in any of these can kill off the little death. So even our most automatic reflexes are not necessary, strictly speaking.

Orgasms are contingent, *Homo sapiens* is contingent, evolution is a contingent development on a contingent planet. And perhaps — as philosopher Alfred North Whitehead once observed — all these things arose in a universe that might have equally been otherwise.

To speak of necessity is usually to speak of possibilities, not certainties — and these are overwhelming enough for us mortals. If not an all-powerful god, Ananke is a cosmic regent, legislating for daily likelihoods. And machines like Fuckzilla are her ministers for the erotic.

Chine

This contingency is vital to understanding Fuckzilla.

First, contingency is important because it is true — and cosmically so. What seems like the adamantine grip of destiny is actually many hands, massaging and nudging. And each of these was massaged and nudged in turn. We are often creatures of blithe certainty, and it does us no harm to recognise the world's muck and flux.

Perhaps some of Intruder's audiences enjoy the fantasy of necessity *because* they are aware of contingency. One of the most persistent masculine tropes is faultless virility: boners that continue for hours. Always hard. And always hard at the right moment. There is a manic tone to macho arousal; a register of hysterical stiffness. It resonates with desperation.

Witness: the *Kama Sutra* recommends drinking 'milk boiled with the testicles of a ram and a goat and mixed with sugar' to help with virility.

Male pornographic actors personify this compensatory priapism — often with the help of drugs — but Fuckzilla and its fellow props do it comfortably. They offer the spectacle of rigid necessity, without the intimidation of another naked man. Put another way: the fuck machines offer the reassurance of anonymous machismo.

But contingency also speaks to freedom, however humble it might be. Without consent, necessity becomes alien — even sexual necessity.

Think of a world governed tyrannically by Ananke; a world of nothing but pure physical and biological necessities. Obviously we cannot remove ourselves wholly from this vision. As philosopher Markus Gabriel notes, our dehumanised world pictures are very much human ones. Still, we can at least fantasise knowingly.

In this imaginary Ananke universe, arousal is possible. Chemical signals are exchanged. Nitric oxide leads to tumescence. There are spasms then jets of fluid. Then, eventually, it all occurs again. And again. And again. Now think of a whole planet of this: just organs periodically pulsing and spilling into one another, until the earth is burned up by the sun. No doubt much of this is truly automatic. No doubt it is also successful: life continues over the generations. But in all of the squelching and heaving, there is no awareness. It is pure happenings.

This is not what sex is like at all, because it is only 'like' something for conscious beings. We exist in significance. What makes sex *sex* is that it means something. And much of this meaning has to do with intimacy, and our willingness to enjoy it. In other words, insofar as the fuck machines are sexy — and they might leave you bored or annoyed — they are so because the performers give themselves over to their trysts. The actresses are not simply vaginas to be filled or rubbed; not simply engorged or lubricated flesh. They are also unique consciousnesses, who consent to unyielding, unrelenting pleasure — or ought to. It is not sexy that the woman is screwed by the robotic dildo. It is sexy that the woman *chooses* to be screwed; that she smiles on her hands and knees, as she readies herself.

This is why these movies dramatise a relationship of sorts, between the model and the personification of Ananke. Because only the model can turn a rubber cock on a camshaft into a story of flirtation and wild abandon. Only the model can make a robot sexual, since only she can allow the thing to fuck her — not vice versa.

In 'Chine', poet Shastra Deo observes the carnage of our urges; the feeling of animal flesh in animal teeth and gullets, which punctuates our intimacy. But there is also a surrender in adoration and lust, which is what makes Fuckzilla pornography and not a documentary about predation on the savannah. If there is acquiescence to helplessness here, it is powerful. 'You bare your throat to the stars,' Deo writes, 'back arches, spine a summit hewn of ivory'.

If I must imagine the actress in the industrial room orgasming, I must also imagine her willingly, powerfully baring her throat like this.

Solidarity

On Paid Sex

I begin with two stories. Or one story told twice. Or
no stories — just two senses of an atmosphere, given a
pleasing form.

They were neat.

They were also quiet, slow-moving, with a lilt in their
accent. But it was their neatness that most struck me:
black hair combed to the right, slacks without creases,
pristine floral shirt. There was effort behind all this: a
daily regimen of washing, ironing, grooming. The labours
behind the simplicity.

I had never visited them before, and I was nervous in
the waiting room. A first time for me.

But they were so exact. Everything about them was
just so, and their private room was very much *theirs*: a
cool palette, with nothing draped or strewn or dropped.
On the wall were a hard-edge painting, three or four

mandalas, and their licence to practice.

They asked about my work, and my children. They had two themselves, of similar ages. We both smiled, spontaneously. The labours behind the simplicity.

Then I stopped smiling. Because I had to tell them what I needed. And what I was paying them for.

Making notes as I spoke, they nodded regularly to let me know they were listening. They asked me to take off my pants, lie on the bed, and make myself comfortable.

I was not comfortable, but I welcomed their trim calm.

Then the doctor snapped on latex gloves, and — still chatting to put me at ease — slowly slid a finger into my arse.

They were neat.

They were also quiet, slow-moving, with a lilt in their accent. But it was their neatness that most struck me: black hair combed to the right, slacks without creases, pristine floral shirt. There was effort behind all this: a daily regimen of washing, ironing, grooming. The labours behind the simplicity.

I had never visited them before, and I was nervous in the waiting room. A first time for me.

But they were so exact. Everything about them was just so, and their private room was very much *theirs*: a cool palette, with nothing draped or strewn or dropped. On the wall were a hard-edge painting, three or four mandalas, and their licence to practice.

They asked about my work, and my children. They had two themselves, of similar ages. We both smiled, spontaneously. The labours behind the simplicity.

Then I stopped smiling. Because I had to tell them what I needed. And what I was paying them for.

Making notes as I spoke, they nodded regularly to let me know they were listening. They asked me to take off my pants, lie on the bed, and make myself comfortable.

I was not comfortable, but I welcomed their trim calm.

Then the escort snapped on latex gloves, and — still chatting to put me at ease — slowly slid a finger into my arse.

Fallen

One of these stories is banal: the stuff of everyday health and well-being. The other is seemingly sordid: the stuff of grim neighbourhoods and twilight rendezvous. What sets them apart?

Sure, prostate examinations are not edgy trysts, or occasions for edging — not for me, at least. But this procedure was *almost* sexual. We had small talk, nudity, lubrication and penetration. Medicine is seen as a sexy vocation, and plenty of straight men enjoy butt stuff. A small study of heterosexual men by Jonathan Branfman and colleagues in *Sexualities* reported that almost a quarter enjoyed anal rubbing and prodding. Put simply, the examination was an intimate moment, involving the touching that typically happens between lovers — touching that some enjoy.

Just as importantly, the medical procedure was not a favour for a friend, or even a gratis public service. My wallet opened not long after my anus. In short: I paid a stranger to put a finger in me. And this stranger was an esteemed professional.

The single word 'escort' changed this dramatically. Someone paid to poke my arse for jollies would no longer be so respected. They would apparently be a lesser creature, to be pitied, mocked, or punished. In short: they would be inferior, with all the sympathies and antipathies this prompts. In the mid-eighteenth century, author Samuel Johnson expressed this superiority with all the moral authority of a Georgian-era gentleman. In his magazine *The Rambler*, he lamented those poor wretches who roamed the night, fucking men. (Men like his buddy and biographer, James Boswell.) For him, these women were dirty, stinking, ugly, often mad. They were seen as 'fallen', and the metaphor is telling. Like the flesh in Plato or Augustine, they were pulled down, away from higher transcendence. Throughout history, the same ideas have been used regularly about those who screw for money: low, mean, base, abject. They all refer to some nether existence, mired in metaphysical and actual filth.

In short, we witness a strange transformation here. Buying and selling medical penetration is wholesome. Buying and selling sexual penetration is nasty. It is terrible to do, and it has equally terrible consequences for everyone involved. If they are not physically ill, they are morally so.

But why?

Prostitute and Other Slurs

Before I answer this question: a brief discussion of the language.

'Prostitute' is an ugly word. Like 'harlot' and 'slut', it typically refers to a shameless woman; a woman exposed, and evilly so. She supposedly has no principles to stop her offering her flesh; no protective layers, literally or figuratively. The word is typically gendered female, though it is used for anyone who is pure availability.

This is why some are still accused of prostituting themselves when they chase wealth rather than ideals. The first century Roman satirist Persius lambasted fellow poets for composing for coins: they fed others' ears, he mocked, and thereby got fed. Dryden's seventeenth-century translation of Persius used 'prostitute' quite specifically. Even lifeless stuff can be slighted in this way, if it falls short of piety. In the sixteenth century, the German reformed theologian Wolfgang Musculus wrote of the prostitute idols in churches, distracting the faithful from the majesty of His creations. A prostituted thing was a common thing, far from sacred. It offered itself too easily. Half a millennium later, this gist remained. The Hungarian author Ferenc Molnár described his own writing as prostitution: first for joy, then for his mates' joy, and then for cash.

There were exceptions to this condemnation. In his sixteenth-century history of England, the Italian Renaissance scholar Polydore Vergil wrote that King Aethelred praised the glory of prostituting himself for his country. Here, the word means devotion; a giving of oneself, without reserve.

But over the centuries, this praise has been rare. Typically, to prostitute oneself is to sully oneself ethically through gain.

Because of this, 'prostitute' is too much the dysphemism. Likewise for 'whore', which has a robust

Germanic register, and which some in the industry have understandably snatched back from grasping misogynists. 'I am a Whore,' writes Veronica Monet, 'and damned proud of it.' I agree that it is wrong to clothe this profession in Pollyanna euphemisms; to pretend respect must be purchased with a fake smile. But these are not words I — the bourgeois philosopher guy — can use comfortably about others. From me, it still smacks of contempt and control.

The recommended phrase is 'sex worker', which is usefully broad, and emphasises labour, not sin or crime. But like the word 'sex' itself, it is also bureaucratically dull: the lexicon of officialdom. 'Sex worker' also suggests an equality that is misleading if not mistaken. While women have no monopoly on this industry, they are the chief sellers, and men the chief buyers. As Sarah Ditum argues in the *New Statesman*, it is deceptive to write of sex work without also writing of gender.

I like 'sexsmith', though the homonymic town and surname do confuse things. ('Sex' in these comes from *seax* — an Anglo-Saxon knife.) This word acknowledges that the work is chiefly about getting off, but also emphasises craft. It speaks to training, standards, and the enjoyable exercise of talent. In this way, 'sexsmith' highlights plural pleasures: of the buyer, but also the seller. 'Much of my satisfaction,' writes sex worker Jessie Sage in *The Pittsburgh City Paper*, 'comes from a job well done.' Similarly, male escort David told *Out* magazine: 'You have sex with men ... sure. But what you're really doing is whatever it takes to make your clients feel like they count — that they're human for that hour or that weekend.' He says this with pride. Trans woman Xoài Pham describes herself as a 'therapist', and lauds her emancipatory role.

Were I more idealistic, I would use 'sexsmith' to convey all this.

But I am not idealistic, and this is not my linguistic sandbox. I am trying to best portray others' experiences.

In an essay for *Kill Your Darlings*, nonbinary writer Vince Ruston observes that two stories dominate here: titillating glamour or horrifying morality tales. Both are partially correct, but partiality can support the most robust lies — those with slim struts of truth to prop them up. 'Sex workers are not a homogeneous group,' Ruston writes, 'and each sex worker has a different experience.' These experiences ought to be respected, and reflected in the language.

So, where possible, I describe what is performed, rather than some generic performer. Otherwise, I use 'sex worker', because those in the industry typically recommend it. I recognise that this is broad and falsely neutral — but my discussion is neither of these. I am writing about adults who consent to sexual services for payment, sometimes because of poverty. They are mostly women. My language does not disguise or distort these facts.

Loathing of the Flesh

So, what is so supposedly monstrous about sex work, prompting Johnson and countless other sermonisers to rave?

The evil cannot be payment for physical labour, as my physician was well and truly using their finger. In fact, even the most desk-bound jobs involve certain muscular and skeletal habits, and not others. All work maintains what

Bourdieu calls a *hexis* in *The Logic of Practice*: a physical
and mental disposition, which realises social values and
ideas. From escorts to physicians, we all labour with our
bodies somehow. The evil cannot be paid intimacy, as my
prostate procedure was textbook closeness. The evil cannot
be harm, since doctors are also under threat. A review in
Occupational Medicine by Ananth Vijendren and colleagues
found physicians suffering from high levels of stress, and
surgeons from needle wounds and musculoskeletal pains.
The point is not that sex work and medical work are
equally dangerous, but that danger need not lead to stigma.

So, corporeality, proximity, or jeopardy — these are
not enough to explain the scent of brimstone that hangs
about sex work. No, paid sex is condemned because it is
paid *sex*.

More specifically, it is vilified because it is neither
matrimonial nor procreative. For conservatives like Kant,
this means it is wicked long before dollars change hands.
It is fucking without babies in mind, and doing so out of
wedlock — everything that dutiful pious screwing is not.
This is why metaphors of lowliness dominate discussions
of sex work: heavy flesh is corrupting ascendant spirit.
The 'fallen' have destroyed the rightful cosmic hierarchy.
They are perverse.

But this criticism is doubly confused. Again, our organs
are not the sanctioned means to some sanctioned end. There
is no evidence that screwing for kicks, companionship, or
rent money is against any divine laws. Indeed, there is
no evidence of a divinity at all, let alone a god who cares
whether or not I charge pegging to my credit card.

Conservatives also tend to gild the lily of matrimony
itself. Countless marriages have been more about wealth,
property, and status than any celebration of godly

union. As Indian sex workers put it in their celebrated manifesto: 'since property lines are maintained through legitimate heirs ... capitalist patriarchy privileges only such couplings.' Within this contract, far too many 'good wives' have been treated merely as wombs, not as the autonomous beings Kant celebrated. And even without earnest baby-making, a wife can become a concubine. In *The Second Sex*, Beauvoir wrote that marital fucking has too often been a service claimed for payment — even if this payment is in food or shelter, not lucre.

So, these orthodox arguments are weak. And perhaps this is because they are often afterthoughts: ethical stretches used to cover up more primal tics and flinches. The traditional condemnation of sex work has little to do with the labour itself; with the exchange of services for money. Instead, it arises from an ancient horror of the flesh in general, and men's fear and loathing of women's flesh in particular. While sex work obviously involves all genders, it has typically been seen as a female job for male clients — and typically *is* this. Overwhelmingly, most in this industry are women. And women are threatening when they are not controlled by their fathers or husbands. As Nussbaum argues in 'Whether from Reason or Prejudice', women's desire is a problem, so sex work becomes a problem. Regardless of sex workers' actual feelings for their clients, conservatives believe the profession liberates noxious female lust, which must be ceased or contained. This is not really about blessed union — this is about patriarchal power.

Male sex workers are often tainted by this same outlook. They are men chiefly servicing men, and queer fucking is seen as a sin or vice; a transgression of the god-given law of heterosexual conception. More importantly, they are not seen as *real* men. Here, the authentically masculine is the buyer, the penetrator, the ejaculator — the one who claims what is his. To be the seller, the penetrated, the swallower? This is seen as feminine; as passively subservient, not actively dominant. A sissy. A fairy. Well into the twentieth century, gay men were understood as women of sorts, as historian George Chauncey notes in *Gay New York*. Put another way, conservatives have a gender hierarchy behind their judgements: the more men seem like women, the lower they are. As sociologist Michael Kimmel observed, living as a 'man's man' essentially means living *against* women.

So, the traditional diatribes against sex work are vague, superficial, or simply misogynistic. They tell us little about the actual business of buying or selling blowjobs or anal play, and more about patriarchy and its shibboleths.

Queer Things

If the problem is not perverse sex for money, perhaps it is the perversion of sex *by* money? In other words: commodification.

In its simplest form, this can be an aristocratic flinch from any paid labour. Since Plato at least, the well-born have sneered at the need to work. In *Sophist*, the Athenian noble famously scoffed at another teacher as a paid chaser of youths. The contemptible part was the pay, not the chase. While Socrates was a seducer of young men, arousing them with his chaste wits, he took no *drachmae* for his performances. Well into the twentieth century, we see old money mocking professionalism in the same way.

But blue-blooded sneers are no help with sex work and its supposed evils. They are a slight against anything that goes beyond amateur dabbling, and slander all of us who work for cash.

A better criticism of screwing for money is broadly Marxist. As the German philosopher noted, commodification is puzzling. The commodity seems very ordinary: as plain and palpable as a naked body on a bed. But it is actually weird, as he observed in *Capital*. In the market, we no longer see work, or the raw materials it extracts and transforms. We see goods with exchange value, abstracted from their human and natural origins. While workers make these products, their worth is understood chiefly through a price. In this way, human beings lose touch with our unique powers. We can no longer see ourselves in a world of our own making; no longer reflect on our existence through a universe we have helped to build. In short: a schism opens between what we sell, and what we are. Marx observed this in his *Economic and Philosophic Manuscripts of 1844*: the more we give to the market, the less we have for ourselves.

More matter-of-factly, we are also alienated by the use and misuse of our skills. Rather than being guided by our own curiosity or talent, we are pushed by financial necessity. And for others' profit, this necessity grows ever faster. It bores minds with tedium and destroys bodies with toil. In *Capital*, Marx describes a juggernaut of capital, crushing workers and their families.

In this way, the sex worker's body can become psychologically distanced from her; can seem like a thing for others' pleasure and profit, rather than her own. Philosopher and former sex worker Yolanda Estes writes of her 'object-like status' on the job, and describes herself taking up 'passive acceptance, false obedience, and alienated execution'. And while fucking for money, the sex worker cannot simply thrust or fist as she pleases; cannot always sigh or laugh spontaneously. She is there to service the client, whether she is turned on or not. 'It was joyless,' Melissa Petro wrote recently in *Vice*. 'I had nothing in common with my clients. Sometimes I hated them.' Similarly, English student 'Sophie' told the *Independent*: 'I pretend to like them, and then get out. Once that hour is done, it's out the door, goodbye.' Over the months or years, this can lead to a protective cynicism, which numbs anxiety but also joy.

By performing lust she does not feel, the sex worker might also support a caricature of women: what might be called the 'fuckdoll' persona. The fuckdoll is not simply lustful, but is lusting after *exactly what men want*. Philosopher Jeffrey Gauthier argues that this can widen the split between how women are sexualised and their actual sexual pleasures. Men's desire becomes the default.

Not surprisingly, clients often feel entitled to enjoy this default. A small study by psychologist Melissa Farley and colleagues reported that men who pay to fuck have less empathy for sex workers, and higher sexual aggression. These clients know that women might only be working in brothels or on the street out of desperation — they are not naive. But these men believe that they deserve to screw, regardless of women's feelings. This is a learned narcissism.

In her essay 'Gasp under Gasp, Sigh behind Sigh', queer sex worker Tilly Lawless portrays a moment of this masculine egotism. She describes a threesome with a client and fellow professional, in which the john is clueless. She writes of the other woman 'holding in her laugh as

I turn a yawn into a moan ... pulling me in to breathe "I love you" against my lips while the client furiously masturbates, oblivious.' Witness that familiar 'oblivious'.

So, even the most gentle or polite men can still be dead to sex workers' feelings. These clients need not be fantasists about these feelings; need not believe these women are genuinely devoted to serving men, as Gauthier worries. Theirs is the more typical vice of the more powerful: they simply do not care.

The juggernaut also capitalises on suffering. Sex work is the last resort for many rejected by their families and communities, or fleeing domestic or state violence. They would not choose the industry if they were not powerless and poor. This vulnerability leads to more vulnerability: to coercion and exploitation. Trafficking flourishes wherever there are people fleeing war or want: from Lebanon, to Italy, to Indonesia. And witness Venezuelan women in Colombian border towns, servicing locals for cash or supplies. Refugee Gabriela told *Voice of America* that she travelled for almost a day to Cúcuta to provide for herself and her two children. She knew exactly what job awaited her, but had little choice. 'This is hell,' she said. Ostracised queer men in Kenya turned to sex work to support themselves and often their families. Martin Kyana, speaking to *Deutsche Welle*: 'I was often beaten up but I had to learn to get back on the street the next day ... to earn more money.'

Transgender sex workers report similar threats. A recent study by economist Christopher Carpenter and colleagues found American transgender citizens to be lower on almost all measures of well-being. They are also at greater risk of assault and murder, which often worsens in the skin trade — especially where it is criminalised.

They are threatened by johns, violent criminals, but also by the police. A transgender woman working the streets in the United States told researchers: 'every time I see a cop I get apprehensive cause I knew I was either going to go to central booking or the nearest hospital'.

For many, these dangers can also combine with conservative clients' homophobia and transphobia. 'There's just so much riding on your femininity and your "realness",' genderqueer sex worker Billie told *Popsugar*, 'that if ever that illusion is broken at any point, they freak out.' As always, precarious masculinity will prop itself up with more precarious others.

Even in safer brothels or agencies, the market can replicate and reinforce inequalities. However 'exotic', workers of colour are often paid lower amounts. Escort Amber Ashton: 'Our rates in the agency were set rates, and my rate was always less.'

The grind for cash can also encourage harm. Annie Sprinkle, a tireless and rightly shameless defender of sex work, writes of 'burnout syndrome' among most professionals. Even if the money is good, it requires toil to earn. Vince Ruston summarises this elegantly:

> Being able to work one night a week and have my rent for the next month secure is far preferable to working three days a week on minimum wage, then going to class another three days, and barely making rent. This is what I tell myself as I tuck a heat pack between my legs and another on my abdomen.

If sex work has its evils, they are economic and political, not spiritual: alienation, exhaustion, cruelty.

Labour

Which is another way of saying: sex work is work. Which is another way of saying it can leave the worker dulled, bitter, tired at best — and exploited and harmed at worst. Marx noted this himself: the logic of prostitution is the logic of *all* commodification. This was echoed by Indian sex workers in their manifesto. 'Our stories are not fundamentally different from the labourer from Bihar who pulls a rickshaw in Calcutta,' they wrote, 'or the worker from Calcutta who works part time in a factory in Bombay.'

As this manifesto also observes, what so often worsens the skin trade is not fucking for dollars, but the poverty that encourages it, or the stigma that still comes with it. A Dutch study by Ine Vanwesenbeeck found that female sex workers in safe, secure employment had similar levels of burnout to female health-care workers. Overwork is a serious problem, but it is a *common* problem: toil and anxiety are harassing, whatever the job itself. As in hospitals and medical surgeries, this is better addressed with occupational health and safety measures than with moral stain or gaol. Vanwesenbeeck also observed that motives mattered. Women who turned to sex work out of desperation were more likely to be stressed and fatigued. In short, the enemy is often penury or trauma, not the labour itself. A placard by protesting German sex workers put this succinctly: 'Fuck the patriarchy — but not for free.'

The vilification of sex workers can often be far more damaging than screwing, stripping or whipping for money. Amy Boyajian describes the gleeful freedoms of being a dominatrix, then her sudden exhaustion and anxiety. 'It wasn't necessarily the work or the clients that left me feeling this way,' Boyajian wrote in the *Huffington Post*. 'The feelings of isolation and loneliness from how I was perceived and treated by others really got to me.' Likewise, former escort Andrea Werhun in *Vice*: 'The shame and stigma of being a sex worker often outweighs the long-term benefits of flexible, well-paying work.' As often happens within persecuted communities, some in the industry have taken up this chauvinism themselves. Witness progressive New Zealand, where some professionals still look down at streetwalkers. One anonymous sex worker told an academic: 'You know — "we're not all wearing fishnets". Well what if we were? You know what is wrong with that if we were all wearing fishnets and stilettos? And what if we all fitted the stereotype — so what?' Hierarchies within hierarchies, with stress rising as status falls.

Alongside this psychological damage are the various dangers of criminalisation, and the withdrawal of rights, protections, and support. Courtesan Sarah Greenmore put it plainly in the *Independent*: 'Keeping our industry in the shadows keeps an unfair power balance in the hands of law enforcement and clients who mean us harm.' This is especially so for marginalised sex workers, who might be forced out of mainstream work by bigotry, then victimised by the selfish and brutal. They deserve workplace and policy reforms, not vilification, prosecution, or religious salvation. As gender and sexuality expert Lauren Rosewarne argues, we need not adore this industry, or find it emancipating — we just need to recognise and reaffirm its workers' autonomy. As *all* industries ought to.

Yes, this labour often involves feigning lust — and so even safe, legal sex work can split psyches. But the skin trade has no monopoly on a schizoid mentality. Think of the doctor, who performs affable ease while fingering the philosopher; the nurse who jokes to comfort the patient before a vasectomy. (I was grateful, but not comforted.) And even more domestically: the cheery but numbed primary school teacher, the calm driving instructor ready to grab the wheel, the charming clerk on his fourth coffee. Labour often asks us to fake it — even the labour of philosophy.

No doubt some men are willingly fooled by the show, believing that all women exist solely to make them come. Misogyny is pathologically deceived and deceiving. But for many johns, the performance is just a performance. For good or ill, this is exactly why they are visiting a brothel, or calling an escort, or pulling up at the curb. They see these workers as the rule's convenient exception: women who will give them what they want. And what do they want? Easier and more immediate gratification, intimacy or entertainment — all without the need for courtship or even kindness. 'Men will be men,' writes Melissa Petro, 'they want a little attention, they want some company, they want an ego boost, they may want to fuck.' In this, johns are typical commodity consumers, with all the alienation this suggests: they seek goods, not labour or its conditions. As always, money loosens or cuts the threads of recognition. This callous fetish will last at least as long as capitalism does, and it touches us all.

Familiarity

It is tempting to seek some novel theory of sex work; to afford some astonishing 'ah ha' moment, which profoundly changes our perception of the trade.

But I ought to resist this temptation. Partly because it can become another egotism: making the profession into a stage for my intellectual agility. Witness my cleverness; smile at my mind, as it pirouettes around these curious abstractions.

More importantly, it is the *familiarity* of sex work that preoccupies me. It is not some startlingly unique job, which tarnishes or polishes the sacred. There is no metaphysical essence of sex here, which can be distilled then sold by the gram. Nobody is selling their bodies or souls. The industry involves erotic, libidinous, and sometimes romantic labour.

Because of this, sex workers are not some exotic cabal, to be shunned for their vices or beatified for their liberations of the spirit. Like most of us, they are workers. They have jobs. I let this banal fact — with all it suggests of autonomy or heteronomy, exploitation or emancipation, pride or shame, camaraderie or individualism — speak for itself.

In lieu of sermons, damnation, or cash, I offer sex workers my solidarity.

Akiko's Boys

On the Reality of Fantasy

Akiko seems nice.

Once a promising classical singer, she now translates between Japanese and Italian. She uses her left-over money to dote on little boys. Aloof to her own wardrobe, she buys an expensive shirt for Shūichi, the son of a more successful soloist. Akiko smiles at the four-year-old's cheeks and ears, and laughs 'warbling, full-throated' as he wriggles out of his new top. Elsewhere, she helps a toddler with his watermelon, poking out the seeds for him. After he chomps the dripping pulp she takes a bite herself, and the boy offers it to her. She is not bothered by his filthy fingers or sticky hands. She finds his simplicity sublime; finds his naivety 'spiritually restoring'. Akiko seems the ideal auntie: generous with her hours, yen — and love.

Akiko also has daydreams about little boys being tortured. Angry after her lover Sasaki stays away longer on a work trip, she guzzles the beers she bought for their date, stuffs her mouth full of crisps, then passes out on the floor. She wakes calm but horny, then the visions begin: of a father smacking his son's face as punishment, then whipping him with a crocodile skin belt and cane, then burning him against corrugated iron, then slitting open his belly, and so on. 'Akiko would often reach the heights of sexual ecstasy ... her pulse beating faster and faster, and her skin streaming with sweat.'

This tale by celebrated Japanese author Taeko Kōno, 'Toddler-Hunting', is both horrific and enlightening. It tells us little about Akiko herself. Like so many of Kōno's stories, this is sexually explicit but only psychologically suggestive. We learn enough to prompt questions, but not enough to answer. Yet Akiko's sadistic dreams are revealing as fantasies. And they are revealing because they are typical in structure if not in content. They demonstrate a great deal about our invented lives — not necessarily about what we want, but about *how* we want it.

We Are Already Imaginary

To begin, a clarification: fantasy is not simply imagination.

Imagination seems otherworldly, but it is actually part of matter-of-fact life — in fact, it helps to create our matter-of-factness in the first place. Think of Akiko watching Shūichi's 'plucky little face', or 'chubby little arms' — she is in no doubt whatsoever that these joys are within her reach. But these perceptions are not immediate, they are the very opposite: mediated. Akiko puts together high-pitched sounds, with dusky colours, with linen smells — and she perceives these as voice, skin, clothes. And she further perceives these as 'boy' in general, and 'Shūichi' in particular.

So, the world is certainly there, but it does not come to us naked, so to speak — we dress existence like Akiko dresses the child. All the world's overwhelming flux is coloured and ordered by our mind.

And it is 'our' mind because we also unify these perceptions with a sense of ourselves. This is what Immanuel Kant, in his *Critique of Pure Reason*, called 'pure apperception': it is not just gathering stimuli into a bundle, but making that bundle ours. 'Only because I can comprehend their manifold in consciousness do I call them together *my* representations,' he wrote, 'for otherwise I would have as multicoloured, diverse a self as I have representations'. In other words, in order for Shūichi to be observed in his new shirt, there must be an Akiko observing: putting together *her* experience of tanned skin, the deep red and blue stripes, and Shūichi's 'bite-sized earlobes'.

Ironically, this apperceptive self cannot be observed, since it is the very basis of all observations. Kant argues that we have no straightforward knowledge of this self, because knowledge asks for thinking *and* some phenomenon to think about. Yet there is no phenomenon of ourselves there, just a ubiquitous sense that we exist — or, put another way: a 'we' sense that existence has for us. 'I am conscious of myself not *as* I appear to myself, not as I am in myself,' Kant wrote, 'but only *that* I am.' We can speculate about this apperception as Kant did. But we can never know it as we know the pages of Kōno's stories: by uniting sensations and thought.

So, we are always bringing a self and world into being, together. And this is a creative deed: the unity does not exist until we invent it. What Kant called 'productive imagination' allows our day-to-day intimacy with the universe.

The imagination also works with space and time.

When Akiko looks at Shūichi, she perceives a whole boy: his face in front of her, but also the back of his head, his calves, his feet in shoes. She cannot actually see any of these, but she quite rightly fills in the gaps.

Experience has taught her that human beings grow in certain ways, and she invents what she cannot sense.

Likewise for the past and future. Akiko buys the shirt, hoping that the little boy will struggle to remove it; that she will watch as his body turns to and fro. Sure enough, this happens: 'Just as she imagined, the child started to twist and turn about,' Kōno wrote, 'wiggling his bottom.' But at the time she makes the purchase, Shūichi is nowhere to be seen. She envisions him, along with everything he might do — and these envisioned possibilities continue when he is right before her. 'She could not go without the chance to watch as he tried to get himself out of it.' With everything we encounter, we add these missing details ourselves: their matter and shape, or what they have done and might do next.

So, creativity allows us to perceive ourselves and the world, and to make sense of this spatially and temporally. There is no innocent consciousness; no naive congress with things. Put another way, imagination need not take us away from everyday experience — this experience is *already imaginary*.

Make-Believe

So, well before Akiko daydreams about torture, she is already imagining: the dark apartment, the 'insects … chirruping outside', and the self that is daydreaming alongside them.

What makes her visions fantasies, strictly speaking, is not that they are simply imagined, but that they are imagined selectively. That is, Akiko perceives that the world is one way — lonely, dull, cold — and then enjoys experiencing it otherwise. She sees a full belly, then imagines it split; she sees stripes on a shirt, and imagines them as burns; she sees her own menstrual blood, then imagines 'red fluid trickling down the child's buttocks'. This is what the English philosopher RG Collingwood called 'make-believe'.

In his *The Principles of Art*, Collingwood noted — with Kant and others — that imagination is part of everyday perception. But he also described the kind of partiality that happens in fantasies. Collingwood put it this way:

> Out of the numerous things which one imagines, some are chosen, whether consciously or unconsciously, to be imagined with peculiar completeness or vivacity or tenacity, and others are repressed, because the first are things whose reality one desires, and the second things from whose reality one has an aversion.

Observe Collingwood's emphasis on desire. In make-believe, we invent things because we *want* to. Akiko's visions arise because she gets off on imagining torture, not because she has actually spied a cruel father outside her apartment. So she puts aside the cracked ice, the empty bottles, the elderly neighbours, the mating crickets, and turns to her dreams.

Fantasies are not defined wholly by truth or falsity. Suppose Akiko once saw a child punished, and this memory worked its way into her daydreams. Her vision would indeed be true, if only partially: the beatings, welts, and cries would be drawn from life. But it would be no less a fantasy for this, because Akiko would still be avoiding her apartment for desire's sake; recalling then, instead of now, to arouse herself. Similarly, Akiko could one day witness this vision. In other words, the daydream would start false and, unfortunately, become true. But on this summer evening, in this Tokyo room, it is a fantasy — because she is enjoying her fancies *rather* than this summer evening, this Tokyo room.

Fantasy is a distinctive way of imagining. In essence, it is an experience that denies much of current experience. And it does so because of pleasure and pain: what is denied is less thrilling — or more odious — than what is accepted. This is why Collingwood called make-believe 'imagination acting under the censorship of desire'. It is a way of refusing and repressing perception, because — and only because — this gratifies desire.

Holiday

Does this mean Akiko desires a little boy tortured?

This is the most contentious aspect of fantasy: it seems to suggest planning. Here, daydreams are seen less as symbolic psychodrama, and more as preparation; as blueprints for the construction of reality. Make-believe becomes a *literal* design and scheme.

American philosopher and psychologist William James once argued that ideas motivate behaviour, and we often treat fantasies similarly. 'Every representation of a movement,' he wrote in *Psychology*, 'awakens in some degree the actual movement which is its object.' In this light, the translator's representations will lead to the actual movements of smacking and whipping.

Violence certainly occurs after Akiko's visions — but the bloodied skin is hers. One evening, she has her boyfriend Sasaki whip her with a pearl necklace. He teases her at first, then beats her; she savours 'the sting and the smart, cracking sound'. But the string breaks, as does the membrane of the encounter. Soon, Sasaki returns from the bathroom with a vinyl rope, used for drying laundry. Akiko becomes horny again. He flogs her with the hooks ('use the jagged bits on me, please ...') until her screams have her neighbour knocking. Akiko forgets her lover and herself, and gives herself to the void — she is like a thing, not a human being. She eventually collapses, and wakes chilled and dazed.

Despite the intensity of these fantasies, Akiko remains as opaque to us as she is to herself — this is part of Kōno's mastery as an author. As critic John Williams put it in *The New York Times*, Akiko 'invites our deep and sustained interest but remains ultimately irreducible.'

Nonetheless, there is enough in Kōno's story to prompt reflection. In her torture fantasies, Akiko is not identifying with the father. She is the boy: scourged, bleeding, crying out. She also hates little girls. She finds them nauseating, their typical 'sickly, white flesh ... etiolated body ... yellowish neck' sickening. In fact, she loathed herself at the same age.

Despite her happy childhood, Akiko always felt monstrous as a girl. She once saw a silkworm pupa in its chrysalis, and thought of herself: 'a filthy, dark form being slowly suffocated by threads issuing out of its own body'. She was relieved to become an adult, if not a woman.

So Akiko's make-believe is more complicated than it appears. She shows no interest whatsoever in harming children like Shūichi — in fact, she typically loses interest in them after one meeting. Instead, she begs her lover to harm *her*. And while Kōno does not explain Akiko's psychology, it seems the character wants to be a little boy — in her daydreams, at least. She sees herself in these cheery, tawny toddlers; sees her ideal beauty and 'infinitely innocent' psyche, given the perfect persona; sees boys, but feminised with menstrual trickles and faux-births. Put simply: the boys are her dream self, personified. If so, then her fantasy is as much masochism as sadism. She wants to see these happy avatars — that is to say, herself — suffer the ecstasy of annihilation.

Akiko's visions reveal that fantasies need not be simplistic programmes or agendas. As Collingwood noted, make-believe certainly involves desire. When we daydream, we are wanting — often earnestly and even aggressively. But what exactly do we want? Kōno's story suggests that we can want a fantasy, without wanting it to happen straightforwardly. 'Desire means not the desire to imagine, nor even the desire to realise an imagined situation,' Collingwood wrote, 'but the desire that the situation imagined were real.' In other words, what is desired is the fantasy *as* a fantasy.

This squares with much of William James's theory of ideas. While he believed they encourage deeds, he also recognised that this was neither simple nor automatic. Ideas often come into conflict: one encourages aggression, the other seeks calm, if not peace of mind; one is selfish, the other altruistic. In such cases, we have to concentrate on one idea and forget the others. 'Drop *this* idea, think purely and simply of the movement,' James wrote, 'and, presto! it takes place with no effort at all.' More importantly, James observed that representations were rarely of bodily movements. We typically think, not of specific muscle twitches or limb flexes — pick up the belt, swing at the child — but of results. 'The action,' James continued, 'must obey the vision's lead.' In other words, we have ends in mind, not means. And the end of Akiko's fantasy is not physical attacks, but the quivering emptiness of her own passive punishment.

This does not mean that Akiko is suddenly an exemplary moral being; that she leaves the reader with a comforting depiction of the mind. Her sexual fantasies are repellant, her life troubling. She might suffer from what psychologists call 'autopedophilia'. Those with this condition are both sexually attracted to children, and to themselves as children. In other words: their sexual orientation is partly internal rather than external, concerning themselves rather than others. In a recent study in *Psychological Science* by psychologists Kevin Hsu and John Bailey, almost half of the pedophiles were also autopedophiles. While this hypothesis might not apply perfectly to Akiko — only men were studied by Hsu and Bailey, and the men identified explicitly as pedophiles — it combines with the story's other details to leave an unnerving impression.

But however pathological, Akiko's fantasies cannot be interpreted as simple wishes. They demonstrate that illusions are often to be enjoyed, not acted out. Within them, we give ourselves over to a personal, placatory universe — then return to workaday reality, just as we left it. Make-believe chiefly affects our experience, not our way of life.

Importantly, this is not about our visions being private.

Privacy concerns our power to regulate information about ourselves; about who can be intimate with us, and how. Philosopher Julie Inness defines privacy as 'the state of the agent having control over decisions concerning matters that draw their meaning and value from the agent's love, caring, or liking.' So, it is less about a withdrawal from public scrutiny, and more about who is in charge of this withdrawal, and why.

Akiko certainly has some control. Her cries might annoy her neighbours, but she keeps her make-believe about little boys to herself. But if she did decide to tell Sasaki about her fantasies, they would be no more or less fantastic for this. Their structure and content would be identical — they would just be known by two people instead of one. While sexual make-believe is often private, because of our social expectations, this is not what makes it make-believe.

The essence of make-believe is a withdrawal of sorts: from immediate experience. Yes, fantasy always arises from a given place and time, with all the specifics this suggests. It is not absolutely autonomous. As scholar Gretchen Jones notes in her essay 'Subversive Strategies', Akiko's fantasies are those of a Japanese woman in the sixties, well aware of her lowly status. But she is toying with gender and its expectations; modifying her impressions. And this modification never becomes fact.

In this, Akiko might be quite ordinary — if not healthy. As psychologists Harold Leitenberg and Kris Henning observe in their paper 'Sexual Fantasy', many so-called 'paraphilic' fantasies are distributed across the normal population. 'The terms *deviant fantasy* and *deviant arousal* are... often misleading,' Leitenberg and Henning write, 'unless linked to deviant behaviour.'

While criminals often imagine their crimes beforehand, these same imaginings are common to many others — others who never realise their daydreams in waking life, and never *want* to. Typically, it takes other traits — including low empathy, hostility to victims, drug abuse — to transition from sexual fantasy to sexual crime.

In short, make-believe can be understood as a virtual holiday from the matter-of-fact, not as practice for it. And if it becomes practice, this is not a failure of illusions — it is a failure of morality.

Rousseauian Perversities

So, fantasies can be dangerous to those fantasised about — think of the succubus, with its fetish of cankered femininity. When illusions guide customs or institutions, they become monstrous. And were Akiko's visions taken literally, they would be criminal plots, not mere libidinal play.

But make-believe can also be used against the daydreamer; used falsely to justify how they are understood and treated. It takes an already simplistic idea of make-believe, and turns it into an essence. In this, it is an existential tyranny: *this is what you are, what you ought to be, and what I will make you.*

This tyranny is reminiscent of Jean-Jacques Rousseau's philosophy. For once, this is not about the Swiss-born thinker's horny peccadilloes or marital vices; not about his lust to be spanked or his arse-flashing; not about his misogynistic contempt for his lover and long-suffering partner, Marie-Thérèse Levasseur. It is not even about his wanking fantasies, which he described as a kind of imagined rape: 'to make any beauty who tempts them serve their pleasure without the need of first obtaining her consent'.

Instead, what most resembles this fetishised sexual selfhood is Rousseau's political philosophy. It is why Isaiah Berlin called the thinker 'one of the most sinister and most formidable enemies of liberty in the whole history of modern thought.'

As Berlin argued in *Freedom and its Betrayal*, Rousseau was caught between two absolute ideals: freedom and authority. The Swiss thinker tried to keep both pure. He did this by defining liberty as what we *would* want, if we knew what was best for us. Thankfully, this 'best' was universal, so all rational beings would want exactly the same things. There was no need for give and take; for negotiation and debate about fundamentals; for the balance of competing and conflicting ways of life — no need to actually do politics, in other words. The citizen simply had to give themselves over to the state — or be forced to. And this force was not selfish or cruel, because it was for the citizen's own sake. 'The evil that Rousseau did consists in launching the mythology of the real self,' Berlin wrote, 'in the name of which I am permitted to coerce people.'

What is most troubling about Rousseau's ideas is not simply their danger — although they are genuinely hazardous notions when combined with authority and force. It is not even his arrogance, abstractly deciding what all rational beings long for. Instead, I am chilled by the philosopher's good conscience.

Rousseau saw himself as a loyal friend to liberty, and was utterly sincere in this. 'I love liberty, and I loathe constraint, dependence,' he wrote in his *Confessions*, 'and all their kindred annoyances.' Throughout his life, he bristled at intimacies and formalities alike; he recoiled from obligations and allegiances. He was a restless soul, who was his best self alone on Ile Saint-Pierre. He was honest and accurate when he wrote in *Reveries of a Solitary Walker*: 'I have never been truly fitted for social life'. Yet Rousseau also had an authoritarian bent, alongside a tendency towards deception, cruelty and pettiness. And it is no coincidence that his works were often sacred scriptures within the Reign of Terror. The Jacobins saw in the philosopher a fervent devotee of moral purity. (Robespierre on Rousseau: 'Divine man! It was you who taught me to know myself.')

When I observe misogynists discussing women, Rousseau's mania comes to mind: glorying smugly in its own goodwill, while authorising violence. Just as Rousseau invented the ideal citizen, much of this is prefaced on the eternal and universal Real Woman, in whose name violation is invited. And this Real Woman — deep in her psyche where only the most profound men know her essence — longs to be fucked. She is as grateful for penis as France's citizens were for the guillotine.

Yes, so-called rape fantasies are real and common. They transcend individual ethics and politics, and occur in every demographic. There are feminists who confess to enjoying visions of 'being ravished', as author and activist Susie Bright put it. Bright remembers rubbing herself to fantasies involving her own sexual assault at knifepoint. She describes this in her essay 'Rape Scenes':

> he kept fucking me with his hands, and I was
> frozen, naked on the sidewalk. He talked to

me nasty, he was arrogant, and he teased the
knife against my nipples. Neighborhood people
gathered; he invited them to take his place. I had
this last fantasy twice, both times culminating in
orgasm.

The great Rousseauian conceit is that these fantasies
justify rape, because to daydream about sexual assault is
to *want* sexual assault. As psychologist Jenny Bivona and
colleagues note in a recent paper for *Archives of Sexual
Behaviour*, this approach even characterised scholarly research for many years. Wish fulfilment was taken literally
by academics: fantasy became a simplistic first draft of
waking stories.

It is nonsense. These explanations forget — or
perhaps deny — the chief difference between rape and
healthy sexuality: consent. 'In a rape fantasy two women
are involved: the character in the fantasy,' Bivona and
colleagues continue, 'and the person who is constructing
the fantasy.' Within the spectacle, a woman is overpowered
and taken forcibly. But behind the spectacle, the woman
herself is depicting every grip or thrust. They are *hers*, by
fiat.

As psychologists Susan Bond and Donald Mosher
report, fantasies can also toy with domination and
submission in other ways. The 'victim' is powerless in
the make-believe, but so is the 'perpetrator', as their
desires overcome them — desires given to them by the
fantasiser herself. The whole enterprise arises from her
free consciousness. 'Erotic fantasies take the unbearable
and unbelievable issues in life,' Bright comments, 'and
turn them into orgasmic gunpowder.'

Because fantasies are never wholly autonomous, care

is warranted here. Liberty only goes so far. Survivors report that the damage of rape just as often enters into their make-believe, along with guilt, shame, grief, and anger. In her memoir *Hunger*, Roxane Gay describes fantasising about the man who raped her. 'I felt nothing at all while having sex, I went through the motions, I was very convincing,' she writes, 'and ... when I did think of him the pleasure was so intense it was breathtaking.' Many characters in Gay's short fiction collection *Difficult Women* seek sexual violence for moments of release. In 'Strange Gods', the narrator orgasms as she is fucked with a wine bottle. 'I felt wretched and low. It was a moment of such perfect honesty I came.' Later in the story, we learn that she was raped by her childhood boyfriend and his gang of mates. Put simply, not all pleasure is triumphant. While Bright's illusions emancipated her, there are no easy and generic remedies for trauma.

What all of these reveries — liberating, terrorising, or both — reveal is that rape fantasies are paradoxical. They freely depict a lack of freedom. In this, they are wishes for consensual rape, which is impossible. And this is exactly what makes fantasies so necessary: they are where impossibility can happen *safely*. They withdraw from the everyday world of means and ends, schemes and executions. Made practical, they become monstrous; they grow into Rousseauian perversities. In the ordinary world, assault is just assault.

If Kōno's tale has any simple lesson it is that make-believe is, at best, an invitation to understand. Beyond this, it offers neither absolution nor permission. It often arises from trauma — it can never justify it. In fact, it justifies nothing whatsoever. Rousseau dreamed up perfectly rational Frenchmen, and then fled to 'the shelter of [his] conscience'. At least Akiko, as she lies drunk on her apartment floor, knows her illusions are her illusions.

Imagining Imagination

Akiko's boys present a challenge to imagination, but not the challenge we might assume.

Akiko's fantasy is difficult because it prompts us to imagine fantasy itself; to more carefully envision what it is to have visions at all.

Imagination has a physical basis, but it is no simple material thing; no sharp hook, with which we might be lashed. As Kant's apperception suggests, much of imagination withdraws from perception — in fact, it allows for perception of 'simple material things' like hooks and bloodied flesh in the first place.

Imagination is also epistemologically fickle. We can imagine truthfully, as we fill in missing details, and remember or predict facts. We can imagine falsely, as we hallucinate, repress, or vainly hope. We can also imagine fantastically, as Akiko does — knowingly erecting a fictional palace in which to play. Imagination has no special affinity with verity; it is 'indifferent to the distinction between the real and the unreal', as Collingwood put it.

So, of all our imaginary ideas, 'imagination' is itself a distinctive intellectual achievement; a concept that requires rigour and finesse to put together. We have to imagine it with all its partiality and mercuriality.

Kōno accomplished this troublingly but compellingly. In Akiko's day-to-day dealings, we see imagination as an ordinary skill: recalling or anticipating events, and completing patchy sensations. We also see imagination as make-believe: inventing experience to suit desire. More importantly, we see how these levels of reality coalesce — or do not. Akiko's psyche moves from fabric stripes to burn marks, from period blood to torture wounds, from Shūichi to victim child. But her psyche does not move from burn marks, torture wounds, and victim child to actual violence against Shūichi or anyone like him. Her psyche just makes a boy *of her*.

This is exactly what Iris Murdoch meant when she wrote about 'moral' looking. Putting aside yet another visual metaphor, Murdoch's point was important: it is an ethical effort to avoid our own egocentric distractions and distortions. Akiko is imagining selfishly. In describing Akiko, the author of 'Toddler-Hunting' was not.

Put another way, Kōno's tale is not make-believe; not pure fantasy. It is a wholly fictional description of sexual intoxication, but it is soberly realistic. It uses imagination to make sense of imagination, and does so with a psychological fidelity alien to fantasists like Rousseau.

Ontologically Nimble

Kōno explores sexual fantasy without her own illusions getting in the way. How might we become equally realistic about make-believe? What qualities make for such a fine witness?

For Aristotle, the ideal soul displayed all the moral virtues, as each was necessary for justice — the good citizen had 'excellence entire', he wrote. But to make sense of fantasy, four excellences seem especially helpful: curiosity, patience, bravery, and perseverance.

Curiosity is an obvious starting-point. This is not the salacious sniffing-out of musk, but the joy of discovery; the willingness to look further than the obvious, and to find this looking an intellectual thrill. Witness the tales of Chinese author Pu Songling, who lived in the seventeenth and early eighteenth centuries. These stories are often erotic, though rarely explicit. There are bizarre fantasies, often involving ordinary mortals with animals or spirits. In one story, a kung fu master takes off his cock, then beats it with a mallet. A perfect emblem of macho vanity, which ends with a hilarious detail of sudden reserve: 'But he refused to try using a knife.' For the Qing secretary and private tutor, the world of flirtation and fucking was less an efficient device for tumescence, and more an encounter with oddness or eeriness. His most recent translator, John Minford, puts it well: 'Sex for Pu Songling is simply one arena in which human behaviour can be observed in all its extraordinary intensity, richness and variety.' Drawing on various folk and literary traditions, Songling displays a connoisseur's eye for idiosyncrasy.

Another virtue is patience. Fantasies are often immediately striking, but not always immediately comprehensible. We can be mistakenly aroused into haste. Freud himself touched on this, informing a correspondent that learning about psychoanalysis meant undergoing psychoanalysis — and this took time. 'Once this has begun,' he wrote to philosopher Heinrich Gomperz, 'it is not so easy to bring it to an end.' But for all his willingness to book multiple couch sessions, the Austrian doctor was hasty. He had an archaeologist's willingness to keep digging, but he always stopped when he believed his spade struck sex.

A better standard-bearer for patience is contemporary

author Adam Phillips — fellow psychoanalyst, but with a far greater tolerance for ambiguity. One of the hallmarks of his work is a circular style: moving from theme to theme in something like a spiral, returning to the same idea with different significance. He paces himself and invites his reader to share his cadence. In his essay 'The Uses of Desire', Phillips draws on Jacques Lacan to distinguish between needs and desires. Needs are straightforward: to know, if not to have. Akiko is hot and needs a cold beer. She could have found herself without a chilled drink in her apartment, but she would still have known she needed one. Desires are vague longings for dreamy chimera. Part of desiring, Phillips says, is the painful pleasure of expectation. And our desires become perverse when we introduce too-easy certainty into this; when we take psychological convenience over the angst of risk. 'Perversion ... is a sacrifice of sorts,' Phillips writes, 'it sacrifices surprise, it sacrifices mutuality, it sacrifices the resonance of the other person and oneself.' If Phillips is correct, what makes Akiko perverse is less her horrific daydreams and more her conveniently casual fucking — she never dares to linger in her desires, but merely nullifies them.

Bravery and perseverance are necessary: the first has to do with facing fear, the other with enduring discomfort. As 'Toddler-Hunting' suggests, fantasies are often horrid — it would be more comforting to read Anaïs Nin's short stories, with their pornographic verve. It takes courage and fortitude to confront make-believe with a steady gaze. This is not prurience — which would mean enjoying what is loathsome — but a kind of steadfastness. Authors like Roxane Gay and Carmen Maria Machado certainly demonstrate this. Their tales are labours of discomfiting illusion — others', and their own.

Another example of these virtues is Nancy Friday, whose *My Secret Garden* introduced millions of readers to women's fantasies. Friday's editorial observations were often psychologically slight, and sometimes just records of her orthodox bigotry — supposedly lesbians are both genders and black men 'reek of sexuality'. But she displayed a laudable willingness to encourage and accept women's fantasies: hundreds of them, archived and catalogued by kink. The panoply is overwhelming. There is a young mother with a newborn who dresses in lingerie, puts in a tampon, then rubs herself to visions of herself — she becomes the small, pale girl, and the dark-skinned man who fingers the girl. There is a lesbian who thinks of herself and her cousin as teenagers, enjoying a threesome with a dog named Anjou: 'I'm fascinated with Anjou's animal maleness; the enormous length of the glistening red, arrow-pointed organ is still exposed'. There is a mother of three who, while screwing her husband, sees herself as a school matron. She lines up the young boys, then jerks them off one by one. And alongside these, countless fantasies of anonymous, vicious, and forced fucking — sometimes by bored Christian wives, sometimes by single swingers.

Friday was criticised for her simplistic celebration of lust; her avoidance of broader issues of privation and domination. *Ms.* magazine famously pronounced: 'this woman is not a feminist'. Hers was certainly an individualistic vision of emancipation, more concerned with therapy than with political or economic change. Still, *My Secret Garden* is a powerful document of sexuality, which treats fantasies as a profound part of existence. And Friday's lack of trepidation or squeamishness is startling: she is interested in truth, not comfort. The connoisseur of make-believe cannot be easily shocked.

To these classical moral virtues, I add an intellectual power: speculation. This is similar to quick-wittedness, in that it asks for psychological flexibility. But whereas *eutrapelia* changes moods with circumstances, speculation changes experience itself: carefully tweaking how we think, feel, and perceive. It is imagination, guided by truth not egotism. No doubt speculation and *eutrapelia* can be joined in practice: I might recall a lover's previous passion to change myself from sulky to horny. Still, these are distinctive mental powers. And what speculation uniquely involves is the knowing and dexterous departure from present fact — not because the fact is unsightly or unpleasant, but because it is not enough to make sense of life. This is why philosopher John Dewey praised imagination, and distinguished it from 'fancy' or 'revery'. 'The healthy imagination deals not with the unreal, but with the mental realization of what is suggested,' he wrote in *How We Think*. 'Its exercise is not a flight into the purely fanciful and ideal, but a method of expanding and filling in what is real.'

Here, the 'real' is the reality of fantasy; the ways in which we use make-believe to pleasure ourselves. As Akiko's daydreams demonstrate, this reality involves a complex panoply: historical gender mores, the symbolism of blood or void, physiological changes because of alcohol or pain, existential projection, and more. To speculate about Akiko's illusions alongside Kōno, we have to imagine all these *kinds* of reality. Speculation asks us to be ontologically nimble, skipping carefully between levels of existence.

We jump this way daily, of course — the great difference is in that little adverb: carefully.

Prince and Lady

On the Meanings of Sex

Our heroes here are a prince and a lady.

They are on a low, wide bed: off-white cotton, chalky grey sides decorated with flowers. (Daisies, perhaps: yellow centres, with white and purple petals.) Her long, straight black hair is pinned back under an orange scarf. His equally dark hair is in a light khaki turban, which matches his rippling robe. Both are wearing jewellery, though hers is more elaborate: nose ring, earrings, necklace, anklets, bracelets, and more. His drop earrings have two pearls. In her powdered-orange fingers, over her powdered-orange palm: a cup, which she is offering him. They gaze at one another, with gentle (almost complacent) smiles.

They seem calm, at ease, sweetly domestic — a genteel married couple, taking tea or wine before visiting one of the many local art studios.

But his cock is half into her, his balls tight. He is kneeling before her splayed legs, brown skin against her pale; free hand on her breast. Her nipples are erect.

There is no ambiguity here: they are fucking. They are also stopping for a quiet drink together, from a fine ceramic cup — while fucking.

I first saw this painting in Peter Webb's *The Erotic Arts*. It was called 'Prince and Lady prolonging intercourse with a cup of tea', and dated to the late eighteenth century. For some years, this was one of my favourite titles: explicit, somewhat absurd, but also oddly wholesome. But it seems Webb got it wrong. The Victoria and Albert Museum describes it simply as 'prince and lady making love' — no steaming beverage to speak of. And if the museum's historians are correct, the miniature was actually made at least a generation after Webb's date, in around 1830. Its opaque watercolours were painted in the state of Guler, in India's western Himalayas.

Suggestions

What does this scene of lovemaking suggest to me?

It suggests patronage. Beginning with India's Mughal rulers, miniatures like this were 'press releases for royalty', as historian Sunil Khilnani puts it. Guler was one centre of Kangra painting, which flourished under the patron Sansar Chand, part of the ancient Katoch clan. Sansar Chand defeated the state's Muslim rulers, and reigned briefly but famously as a lover of the arts. And often, these arts were of lovers. Scenes of nobles or gods screwing — frequently Krishna and Radha — were common. Gazing at these was a *bona fide* aristocratic pastime. One painting has the *maharaja* idling regally in his court: puffing from a *huqqa* in his cameo pink robe, looking at paintings of pretty women. A century after

the king's death, civil servant BH Baden-Powell reported
the maharaja's 'fine collection' and legacy as a patron
— he did not, alas, report on whether the erotica was
enjoyed by British colonials. (Historian Robert Aldrich:
'Colonisers made it their business, at least in theory, to
attack vice.')

It suggests rule. To stop and sip from a porcelain cup;
to take one's time with lovemaking, with neither fear
nor distraction; to do so in a clean, spacious bedroom,
with decorated panelling and lush cushions; and to see
oneself as both the subject and object of such paintings,
an amorous noble and aesthetic connoisseur — such is
the ruler's privilege. In short: our horny couple are rich.
Money and power were also behind the painting itself.
Kangra was supported by the exploitative class relations
of northern India. There was neither the Katoch dynasty
nor Sikh empire — which overthrew the Katochs —
without commoners to fill their coffers. And how did
the Victoria and Albert Museum get this painting? A gift
from Major RG Gayer-Anderson and Colonel TG Gayer-
Anderson, twin British officers — one of whom was an
administrator in Egypt. That is to say: the artwork came
courtesy of empire.

It suggests virtue. Vatsyayana's *Kama Sutra* was
written at least fifteen centuries before this scene was
painted, but it was still read by those with the education
and leisure to read. Translated into Persian during the
earlier Mughal reign, this book was enjoyed alongside
other Indian and Muslim erotic texts. The *Kama Sutra*
describes the good wife's conduct in detail. She will go
plainly while her husband is away, wearing just enough
to show she is married. But 'when going to make love,
she adorns herself with jewellery, fragrant oils of various

flowers, all kinds of powders and bright clothes.' Here, the lady shows that the prince is her only man; that she is loyal and faithful. (She may not be. But she is *showing* this.) For his part, the prince is also well groomed, perhaps trimming his nails and whiskers every fourth day, and keeping his armpits clean. Both he and his lover are calm, a theme common to Hindu and Muslim erotic art — what British Museum curator Imma Ramos calls an 'aestheticised lifestyle'. And behind this etiquette? Ethics. This is as much about right conduct as good manners. The *Kama Sutra* makes clear that both lady and prince ought to be committed to *kama* — pleasure and also its patron god — without wasting money or behaving viciously. 'Man has a lifespan of one hundred years,' the *Kama Sutra* says. 'This time should be parcelled out in so pursuing the three ends of life ... that they do not interfere with each other.'

It suggests cosmology. In Hinduism, sex can be more than casual rubbing or even dutiful baby-making. Each of the three major male gods — Brahma, Shiva, Vishnu — has a female lover, and their lovemaking can be as cosmological as physical. In this vision, mortal bodies become avatars of a sacred universe. The *Brihadaranyaka Upanishad* describes a woman as a temple or altar. 'Her vulva is the sacrificial ground; her pubic hair is the sacred grass,' it says, 'her labia major are the Soma-press; and her labia minor are the fire blazing at the centre.' The esoteric *tantra* cult, which originated between the sixth and eighth centuries, sees sex as especially pious. While moderate tantric schools treat this symbolically, others are more literal: seeing cum and period blood as sacraments, often to be swallowed. By the time of our amorous couple in the nineteenth century, *bakhti* was more common than *tantra*:

a movement of devotion, which sat comfortably alongside Sikhism and Islam. But even if the prince and lady are neither tantric nor *bakhti* adepts, their slow, ritualised sex suggests a belief common to Indian philosophy and faith: that screwing can be reverential, not profane. 'Sensuality continued to keep its foot in the door of the house of religion; the erotic,' writes Indologist Wendy Doniger in *The Hindus*, 'was a central path throughout the history of India.'

It suggests beauty. From her rounded arse and arching back, to his sweeping eyebrows and delicate hand. The burnt orange of her skin and scarf, and the curtains above; the varied greens of his flowing robe; the fuchsia pillow supporting her left leg. The prince and lady are idealised in form and colour — impossibly large eyes, seemingly impossible contortions — but they are neither lifeless nor cartoonish. Their genitals are subtly shaded to suggest shaved hair, without distracting from the crisp lines. His penis is humble — no Japanese *shunga* monster cocks here. This is more about the intimacy of their gaze than about their bits. 'Kangra art is the language of human love,' wrote Indian civil servant and historian Mohinder Singh Randhawa in the sixties, 'intimate, ecstatic and passionate.'

These are just a handful of the ideas prompted by our horny couple. They do not exhaust the painting, or the fucking in the painting. Instead, they spotlight just a little of the scene's vast background. To think about the prince and the lady, for even a moment, is to be overwhelmed by significance.

Put simply: sex is profusely meaningful. It points beyond itself, to a variegated world.

Hole, Ooze, Gash

For much of the modern era in Europe, it seemed the relationship between sex and the world was the other way around: almost everything was about fucking. The most popular portrait of the mind was from Freud, whom literary critic Harold Bloom rightly called 'the most suggestive myth maker of the last century'. The Austrian doctor was an unreliable theorist, but a fine author and artist — he took our bizarre psychology seriously, and gave it powerful pictures and stories. And what was behind this drama, for him? The libido.

In *A General Introduction to Psychoanalysis*, Freud wrote that almost all the symbols in our dreams are sexual. He also observed that many of our mythic symbols are the same: references to genitals, or genital urges. In fact, language itself was once sexual, he said: speech was originally for calling lovers. So *all* symbols arose in a world created by the 'ancient conditions' of desire. And what of art, like the Kangra miniatures? Freud certainly thought fiction was a way to daydream while awake, offering 'a liberation of tensions in our minds', as he put it in 'Creative Writing and Day-Dreaming'. It gave us the small thrill of beauty plus the larger one of impossible satisfactions made possible. Freud wrote little of painting and sculpture, but treated Leonardo and Michelangelo's works as literature of sorts: texts to be examined like dreams for their sexual clues. When trying to crack any artistic code, the Freudian password was always 'loins'.

In this light, a casual Freudian analysis of the prince and lady turns their bedroom into a freakish orgy; a menagerie of genitals. The bottle? A vagina. Doorway, flowers, jewels? Vaginas. Hat? Penis. Water jug? Penis.

And so on: cocks and pussies, all the way down. If this sex is a text, the psychoanalytic subtext is — sex. Swap 'painting' for 'dream' here, and you have Freud's approach: 'The great majority of symbols in the dream are sex symbols.'

It is no surprise that Freud saw sex everywhere: for him, the libido was the steam in the mind's engine. It is also no surprise that generations of psychologists, philosophers and other critics have rightly lambasted the doctor for his reductionism: turning the richness of humanity into the poverty of a single longing.

Philosopher Simone de Beauvoir pointed out that sex is not somehow more primal than labour or the other demands of survival. Yes, the body is fundamental — but the body is not wholly sexual. And this body always exists within a meaningful whole; a tangle of self and other, 'I' and world. 'The hole, the ooze, the gash, hardness ... are primary realities,' she wrote in *The Second Sex*, 'and the interest they have for man is not dictated by the libido, but rather the libido will be coloured by the manner in which he becomes aware of them.'

And precisely because sex occurs in this world beyond sex, Freud's ideas were very much of his time and place. Social psychologist Erich Fromm noted that the Austrian thinker's outlook was more about middle-class Viennese society than any universal theory of humanity. Sex was a common bourgeois anxiety, and Freud's 'science' meant locating this in some basic substance. So the doctor saw sex in all symbols, not because he had hit upon eternal truths, but because he was a modern bourgeoisie making a mythos from his own milieu.

Perhaps more surprising is that Freud never discussed sex *as* the symbol. In his universe, most things meant genitals and their urges — but what do genitals and their urges mean?

Against Freud, what the prince and lady suggest is this: sex is richly meaningful. A single couple, in a single tryst, in a single painting — this is enough to evoke fundamental concepts: political, ethical, metaphysical, aesthetic.

The Meaning of Meaning

A quick interlude on terminology. When I write of meaningful sex, I am not referring to so-called 'meaningful sex'. This is a popular phrase, but it is misleading philosophically.

'Meaning' is a dense word — it stuffs a great deal into its semantic luggage. It is used in several ways, some contradictory. Witness the painting of our prince and lady. Its 'meaning' can include: what it arises from (nineteenth century northern India) or leads to (aristocratic leisure); what it depicts (fucking), suggests (esoteric Indian philosophy), or expresses (elegant intimacy); or simply what I personally associate with it (black tea and halva). Some of these meanings are public, others private. Some are sociological, others psychological. Yes, we do have a more general idea of meaning: an explanation of how something points beyond itself, to use philosopher David Cooper's definition. But this pointing is done in various ways.

In short, 'meaning' has a lot of meanings. When I say the erotic Kangra painting is meaningful, I mean it in this broader way: thick with significance, and many *kinds* of significance.

The common phrase 'meaningless sex' is a far narrower use of the word 'meaning'. It refers chiefly to what the lovemaking arises from, and expresses: romance. Meaningless sex lacks personal proximity — our bodies are close, but not our selves.

Yet sex is never meaningless, strictly speaking. Nothing that exists for us is without meaning. As soon as we encounter or envision anything, it has some significance for us, in Cooper's sense: it points beyond itself, and invites explanation. Witness the seemingly meaningless sex in Carmen Maria Machado's short story 'Inventory': it means, among other things, loneliness. The seemingly meaningless sex in James Baldwin's *Another Country* means, among other things, American race relations. ('In Harlem ... he had merely dropped his load and marked the spot with silver.') The seemingly meaningless sex in Robert E. Howard's Conan tales means, among other things, that the barbarian is the manliest of manly men who can satisfy strangers with his panther-like, lion-like, tiger-like, grizzly-like, cobra-like manliness. *Homo sapiens* lives in and through the gist of things — we cannot help it. As anthropologist Clifford Geertz wrote: 'Man is an animal suspended in webs of significance he himself has spun.' These stay sticky, even during the most casual one night stands.

So, our prince and lady are fucking, and this is full of meaning. But this is not necessarily 'meaningful sex' — they might be strangers, coming together for a single afternoon. Then perhaps she returns to her husband's estate to tend 'charming plots of musk rose and gooseberry', and her lover to his 'mock-fights with wild jasmine flowers'. Far more interesting than their promiscuity is its general significance: the universe of possibilities that girds their naked actuality.

Equiprimordiality

We often try to shrink this universe of meaning. Despite sex's suggestiveness — or perhaps because of it — we grip a handful of familiar meanings. Sex becomes merely sin or vice, procreation, instinct or will, or some other neat idea.

The problem is not that these notions are necessarily false. There are biological urges, however fungible into stiletto heels or furries. While I reject 'sin' as a mistaken and misanthropic concept, there can certainly be vice and virtue. And fucking is part of our species' procreative need — for now, at least. The problem is that these notions are not enough. As Freud's manias demonstrate, a single basic concept rarely does justice to the diversity and specificity of existence.

This is why German philosopher Martin Heidegger introduced the concept of 'equiprimordiality' in his *Being and Time*. We cannot make sense of logic of everyday life without certain fundamental ideas, but no one of these is prior to the others. For Heidegger, we are always with others in a world of relevance, and alongside our tools; always pulling along a past, towards a future; always in a given 'here' relative to some 'there'; always in a mood that shifts perception and passion; and so on. This is why he wrote of Being-in-the-World, instead of just beings. (English translations of Heidegger are filled with hyphens: he was trying to knot together notions we routinely cut apart, and our language is clumsier with compound words than German.)

For this reason, Heidegger was sickened by Freud's works. The psychiatrist Medard Boss introduced him to the Viennese doctor's original writings. The philosopher shook his head throughout — the reading, Boss said of Heidegger, 'made him literally feel ill'. While Heidegger's criticisms of Freud were numerous and sometimes esoteric, one stands out: the father of psychoanalysis kept reducing humanity to drives, or other seemingly scientific stuffs. The Freudian picture was one of physical necessity: creatures pushed to do things by the libido, never pulled along by their own purposes. Heidegger took issue with this reductionism. 'The determining factor is not an urge ... urging me from behind,' he told Boss during a holiday together in Sicily, 'but something standing before me, a task I am involved in, something I am charged with.'

Like Jean-Paul Sartre after him, Heidegger overestimated meaning and underestimated biology, but he was correct about Freud. The doctor ignored our need to interpret the world and ourselves. We might not do this consciously, but we always have ideas of what things are, what they mean, and what all this is worth. And these ideas are lived, not simply thought; they are tendencies of perception and feeling, as well as intellect. Hence Heidegger's rhetorical question to Boss: 'Is the human being present within the total construct of Freudian libido theory at all?'

Freud denied the significance of sex because he denied the significance of existence. Sex simply *was*, because life simply *was*. And how, in the Freudian universe, might we say otherwise? All is libido. In a beautifully circular work of reason, Freud chose to cut away those parts of humanity that gave the lie to his cutting away.

But Freud is only one example of this, and more notable because he was progressive in other ways: daring to take sex seriously, along with our workaday psychodramas. The expanse of our libidinous, erotic and romantic lives is regularly corralled. And even those who think profoundly about love and lovemaking can be as narrow as they are deep; can push aside equiprimordiality in favour of a single shiny idea.

My Shiny Idea

And what is *my* shiny idea? Abstractly, I recognise that sex is one thread among threads. But I also reach for the gleaming filaments and miss those behind.

Take our lady. With her untroubled smile and unhurried gaze, she seems perfectly at ease. Legs wide apart but otherwise still, she is an ideal unity of horniness and poise, tumescence and meditation. Perhaps she reads the *Kama Sutra* or has it read to her, and knows the sixty-four arts of sex and the subsidiary arts including 'enamelwork ... teaching parrots and mynah birds to talk ... knowledge of dictionaries ...' She is educated, beautiful, well-dressed — and has a strong libido. Perhaps the lady is also familiar with *The Perfumed Garden* in Arabic or translation, and knows her prince is one of the few meritorious men. When he nears her, 'his member grows, gets strong, vigorous and hard; he is not quick to discharge, and after the trembling caused by the emission of the sperm,' wrote Muhammad al-Nefzawi, 'he is soon stiff again.' So, our lady is arousing, aroused — and so very grateful.

But this is as much *my* fantasy of her happiness as it is hers. She might simply be a painter's patriarchal fiction — and mine.

The *Kama Sutra* emphasises the importance of a woman's orgasm, telling the good man to help her come before he does. This is obviously far more generous than so many official Christian tracts about marital duty. But the *sutra* also suggests how to drug and rape a maiden, or how to take someone's wife by arresting and gaoling her husband. Sure, Vatsyayana sees these as the lowest of low unions, and celebrates 'mutual love' as the highest. But, ever the pragmatist, he sees violently misogynistic marriage as better than no marriage whatsoever.

Likewise for *The Perfumed Garden*. It praises the good lover's foreplay, and mocks the bad lover for his selfishness, weakness, and clumsiness. But it also lauds a wife who is more her husband's victim than equal:

> She speaks and laughs rarely, and never with-
> out a reason. She never leaves the house even to
> see neighbours of her acquaintance. She has no
> woman friends, gives her confidence to nobody,
> and her husband is her sole reliance.

This is a portrait of abuse, not of marital partnership.

Yes, the *Brihadaranyaka Upanishad* portrays the woman as a temple; as a living symbol of the sacred. Yet she is not even safe, let alone respected as an autonomous human being. It recommends bribery and physical violence if she refuses sex after her period, when she is 'the most auspicious'. If coins or other gifts will not work, 'he should beat her with a stick or with his fists and overpower her'.

Again, these are ancient texts. The *Brihadaranyaka Upanishad* was written over twenty-five centuries before the anonymous Kangra artist painted our prince and lady. Guler of the nineteenth century was not third century Pataliputra, where the *Kama Sutra* may have been written. It was not fifteenth century Tunisia, where Nefzawi reportedly wrote his manual. And the subcontinent was no tidy museum exhibit, with neither change nor conflict.

Still, these were popular erotic texts for colonial-era readers, because they celebrated popular values. Their patriarchal ideals were very much the status quo, whether among Hindus, Sikhs, Muslims, or the invading British. As sociologist Jyoti Puri argues in her essay 'Concerning *Kamasutras*', both classical and colonial India upheld 'the marginalisation and regulation of women and their sexualities, the centrality of the wealthy male citizen'. And Indian women were doubly marginalised: as female, and as foreign. The 'liberated' maidens who laboured and slept with Orientalists like Richard Burton were not part of polite British society. These *bibis* — a title that meant 'miss' to Indians but 'mistress' to the British — worked in nurseries, studies, boudoirs. But they were not welcome as guests in drawing and dining rooms. They were, as Katie Hickman puts it in her popular history of British women in the subcontinent, 'an amenity to be enjoyed in private'.

India was not more misogynistic than elsewhere. But it certainly was misogynistic. And this alone ought to give pause to any exotic, erotic visions; ought to dull my shiny ideas. Sex is prodigiously meaningful, and we ought to be wary of clinging to those meanings that are most conveniently comforting or flattering to us.

Against Reductionism

So, what approach to sex am I endorsing here, through our prince and lady?

This is certainly not pessimism, which confuses the true with the uncomfortable or unattractive. Think of Arthur Schopenhauer, who saw love as nothing more than the instinct to make babies. For Schopenhauer, I do not *really* adore my wife as my wife; for her very distinctive self. No, this is just my spermatozoa seeking an egg. And likewise for the prince and lady: they are just life, twitching and convulsing to make more life. 'The ultimate purpose behind all love-affairs, whether played in sock or buskin,' he wrote, 'is nothing less than *the composition of the next generation.*' Philosophically, this was not a redefinition, this was a refusal. Schopenhauer could not — or perhaps would not — make sense of romance *as* romance. This allowed the German philosopher to dismiss love as nothing more than another painful and vulgar attachment to a painful and vulgar universe.

And it is no surprise that a nervous, suspicious bachelor failed to give romance its dues. He was the needy child of a distant mother — Bryan Magee describes Johanna Schopenhauer as 'one of those brittle, socially oriented personalities who are almost totally devoid of true feeling'. After she threw him out of her house in 1814, they did not see one another again. Schopenhauer never recovered from Johanna's rejections; never achieved intimacy with women or men.

Biography is not philosophy, but Schopenhauer's life clearly guided his ideas. 'Lurking beneath his notes are his metaphysical views on gender and sexuality,' Peter Lewis writes in his biography of the philosopher, 'thinly covering his bitterness towards his mother.' For Schopenhauer, it was better to explain away romance as pure will than to consider himself lacking in genuine goods.

The German thinker was as nasty in life as on the page, but he was lending his eloquent voice to a more general prejudice: that the shocking, grievous, or ugly is somehow more genuine than the comforting or celebratory. This often arises from something like sour grapes: the meaning of something is determined by our need to avoid needing it. This, in turn, leads to a shallow and narrow idea of existence. For purely psychological reasons, we look for the worst in sex and sexuality — and we conveniently stop searching when we find it.

I am also not calling for political simplification: seeing the prince's male domination as the *only* sexual significance. Yes, the painting's milieu was patriarchal — but this does not exhaust its significance.

Feminist author Andrea Dworkin famously said that all straight fucking is dehumanising, and that women who get off on this are suffering from false consciousness. Importantly, Dworkin was not against sex — this idea is a caricature of radical feminism. She celebrated erotic coupling in her essays and fiction. Instead, Dworkin was arguing that sex with men in patriarchy is always objectifying for women; it treats them as things, not human beings. These 'occupied women will be collaborators,' she wrote in *Intercourse*, 'more base in their collaboration than other collaborators have ever been: experiencing pleasure in their own inferiority'.

The problem with Dworkin's theory is that it silences the voices of actual women, who enjoy screwing without being turned into nothing more than tools; into equipment, owned and used thoughtlessly by men.

Writing about Dworkin and her comrade Catharine MacKinnon, Nussbaum observes in 'Objectification': 'they rarely go further, looking at the histories and the psychologies of individuals'.

Applying this to our Kangra painting, there is no denying the patriarchal cultures of nineteenth century India; no denying that our prince had more powers and freedoms than our lady. But as they do today across the world, women in Guler negotiated men's domination variously — and not every relationship was dominating. Historian Padma Anagol argues that we ought not accept a 'passivity model' of Indian women. 'The women's movement of the nineteenth century studied in its own terms,' Anagol writes in *The Emergence of Feminism in India*, 'shows that … women were … creating roles for themselves that often differed from male perceptions and aspirations for them.' Similarly, historian Tanika Sarkar notes the 'everyday acts of defiance by women, in their secret transgressions' and elsewhere. These were not the very public conflicts around gender that arose in the Victorian era, but they are worth recognising. Indologist Wendy Doniger emphasises the 'subjective dignity' of women in Raj India, respecting their sensibilities and choices, however troubling to us. Her point can be generalised to sex: intimacy is not somehow beyond politics or economics, but it cannot be reduced to politics either. We do not know exactly what this fictional lady was thinking or feeling — but we do know consciousness is not merely the mark of an era's stamp.

Sex is too complicated to mean any one thing, and we ought to be suspicious of simple interpretations — others' or our own. Reductionism always falsifies some truth, whether as Freud's reduction of life to libido, or

Dworkin's reduction of pleasure to brutalised complicity. Witnessing carnality, we ought to ask: what *else* might this mean? And more specifically: what might my own feelings be disguising or distorting?

Attentive Pause

I offer the prince and lady as symbols of an attitude.

Even if they speak to real lives in northern India, I know little about their psychology. Perhaps they are dualists, celebrating spirit's beatification of matter. Perhaps they are monists, who see all things as the one dynamic energy. Perhaps they are libertines who care nothing for abstraction. Whatever their ideas, they exemplify a kind of passionate poise. They are not vilifying their desires; not making lust monstrous. Theirs is not a life-denying asceticism. They are practicing sublimation: making their needs more graceful. In their stylised lovemaking, the couple are consciously putting reflection ahead of reflex.

This is a beautiful shorthand for the beginnings of philosophy. We ought to approach the meanings of sex like the prince and lady fuck: enthusiastically, but with attentive pause.

Generous Promiscuity

What I Read to Write This

Literature seems horny, even when the pages are Augustine-chaste. We speak of promiscuous readers, flitting from book to book. Reading is often described as 'intimate', as if the author themselves were at our fingertips. And if not the author, then some Other: a stranger or ourselves, to whom we reach through the words. This is not purely cognitive; not some ethereal thought. We *feel* words. Virginia Woolf, writing to her lover Vita Sackville-West: 'Love is so physical, & so's reading'. For many of us, the eroticism of text can be more prosaic but no less powerful: we first learned about fucking from books, shaking torchlight helping us skim to *that* scene.

But the written word has one added virtue: readers are rarely jealous. What we adore or at least find arousing, we want others to enjoy too. The philosopher Bernard-Henri Lévy once remarked that Sartre screwed his girlfriend Bianca, but the real climax was writing about it to Beauvoir afterwards. This certainly gets to the orgiastic aspects of literature; the way its pleasures are heightened in the giving. With words, my relationships feel more complete when I offer them to others. This is not out of saintliness, but out of a more daemonic urge: I get off on your getting off.

So, allow me to share my pleasures.

The first epigraph comes from Iris Murdoch's *Metaphysics as a Guide to Morals* (Penguin, 1993). Murdoch was an unfashionable philosopher, daring to chase the Platonic Good in an age of utility. She wrote and thought beautifully. The second is from John Minford's translation of Pu Songling, *Strange Tales from a Chinese Studio* (Penguin, 2006), which I discuss here and there. An enormously entertaining compendium of gags, horrors and absurdities.

The Classroom

I came to Frank Herbert's *Dune* (Gollancz, 2011) in middle age — too late to be overwhelmed by its rich world and psychological nuance, but not too late to be impressed. Merleau-Ponty, *The Phenomenology of Perception*, translated by Colin Smith (Routledge and Kegan Paul, 1970). A modern classic, which rightly brought the body into philosophy — though not as pure physicality. I believe I pilfered my father's edition, still holding together after fifty years.

Irving Singer's categories come from *Sex: A Philosophical Primer* (Rowman and Littlefield, 2001). An enormously helpful work, as lucid as it is progressive.

I cannot remember when I first read DH Lawrence's

Lady Chatterley's Lover (Penguin, 1999), but I have never been tempted to go back. Oddly joyless for such a sensual novel. The same cannot be said for Phillip Roth's *Portnoy's Complaint* (Vintage, 1995), which is as funny as it is grotesque — and, ultimately, sad.

Always read Deborah Levy. *Hot Milk* (Hamish Hamilton, 2016) is a fine way to begin. Not having read Marlon James before, I cannot say if *Black Leopard, Red Wolf* (Hamish Hamilton, 2019) is typical. Painfully macho at times, it is also a feverish fantasy world, written with grit and lyricism.

With its long analysis of Freud, Shulamith Firestone's *The Dialectic of Sex* (Paladin, 1972) is somewhat dated intellectually. It is also naive about liberation through technology, which has become more libertarian than communitarian. Still, Firestone's work is politically radical and proudly erotic. Joseph Brodsky's *Watermark: An Essay on Venice* (Penguin, 1992) is by no means radical, but it is certainly erotic: the kind of liveliness Firestone was celebrating.

Jeanette Winterson's *Oranges Are Not the Only Fruit* (Vintage, 2014) is a moving coming-of-age story, which reveals the harm done by conservative shame — but also the joy of fucking without eternal love. Speaking of joy, Alice Tarbuck's poem 'Mary Godwin Shelley's Second Wife' is from *We Were Always Here: A Queer Words Anthology*, edited by Ryan Vance (404 Ink, 2019). 'Sentimental Education' comes from Zadie Smith's *Grand Union* (Hamish Hamilton, 2019).

The study of sexual thoughts and their frequency is by Terri Fisher, Zachary Moore, and Mary-Jo Pittenger: 'Sex on the Brain?: An Examination of Frequency of Sexual Cognitions as a Function of Gender, Erotophilia, and Social Desirability', in *Journal of Sex Research* 49 (2011), 69–77.

Catherine Millet's *The Sexual Life of Catherine M.* (Serpent's Tail, 2002) is translated by Adriana Hunter. Among other things, it is a portrait of a well-respected authority giving up their authority (though not respect) for kicks. David Halperin's articulate and elegant 'What is Sex For?' is from *Critical Inquiry* 43 (2016).

I read James Baldwin's *Another Country* (Penguin, 2001) for the first time only recently. Without a doubt, it is one of my favourite novels: as if Henry James were writing post-war urban queer fiction. A little claustrophobic at times, but brilliant nonetheless.

An excellent overview of philosophers on sex is Alan Soble, 'A History of Erotic Philosophy', *Journal of Sex Research* 46 2–3 (2009), 104–20.

For all my criticisms, I will never tire of Plato. All my references to his works are from *Plato: The Collected Dialogues* (Princeton University Press, 1996), edited by Edith Hamilton and Huntington Cairns. These are well laid out and translated, though Plato can always be found quickly and for free electronically.

Chrysippus' praise of Diogenes is from Plutarch, *Moralia*, Volume XIV (Loeb Classical Library, 1976), translated by Harold Cherniss. Epictetus' discussion of fucking as a 'defeat' is from his *Discourses*, Book II (Loeb Classical Library, 1925), translated by WA Oldfather. Seneca's letter to his mother Helvia is from *Moral Essays*, Volume II (Loeb Classical Library, 1932), translated by John W. Basore. For his neat description of the Stoics, see Diogenes Laërtius' biography of Zeno in *The Lives of Eminent Philosophers*, Volume II (Loeb Classical Library, 1925), translated by RD Hicks. The biography

of Epicurus is from the same volume. I was also guided by
Tad Brennan's 'Epicurus on Sex, Marriage, and Children',
Classical Philology 91 4 (1996), 346–52. Lucretius' *On
the Nature of Things* (Loeb Classical Library, 1924) is
translated by W. H. D. Rouse, revised by Martin F. Smith.
My Plotinus is *Enneads* (Loeb Classical Library, 1988),
translated by AH Armstrong. The quotes are from Volume
VI, V, and III respectively, and Porphyry's blunt judgement
of Plotinus is from the first volume.

Obviously, I am something of a Loeb fanboy. Their
dual texts (ancient language on one side, English on the
other) are enormously helpful, and the volumes themselves
are handsome. I read many through my university's
electronic subscription, but I buy them second-hand
whenever I can.

Augustine's *Against Julian* (2004) can be found in the
Fathers of the Church Series, published by the Catholic
University of America Press, and translated by Matthew
Schumacher. As with all of the church fathers, there are
also plenty of electronic translations. Alan Soble's essay
was helpful: 'Correcting Some Misconceptions about St.
Augustine's Sex Life', *Journal of the History of Sexuality*
11 4 (2002), 545–69.

I only have an electronic edition of Aquinas' mammoth
Summa Theologica (Burns Oats and Washbourne, 1917–
1925), translated by the Fathers of the English Dominican
Province. Should you wish to enjoy your sinfulness with
imitation leather, there are also handsome sets of five or
twenty-two volumes. On Aquinas, I found John Giles
Milhaven very instructive: 'Thomas Aquinas on Sexual
Pleasure', *The Journal of Religious Ethics* 5 2 (1977),
157–81.

On Ficino: Ardis Collins, 'Love and Natural Desire

in Ficino's Platonic Theology', *Journal of the History of Philosophy* 9 4 (1971), 435–42; Katherine Crawford, 'Marsilio Ficino, Neoplatonism, and the Problem of Sex', *Renaissance and Reformation* XXVIII 2 (2004), 3–35; Wouter Hanegraaff, 'Under the Mantle of Love: The Mystical Eroticisms of Marsilio Ficino and Giordano Bruno', in *Hidden Intercourse: Eros and Sexuality in the History of Western Esotericism*, edited by Hanegraaff and Jeffrey Kripal (Fordham University Press, 2008), 175–207.

Denis Diderot's celebration of wanking is in *Rameau's Nephew and D'Alembert's Dream* (Penguin, 1966), translated by Leonard Tancock. *Philosophy in the Bedroom* is from Marquis de Sade, *Justine, Philosophy in the Bedroom, and Other Writings* (Grove Weidenfeld, 1990), translated by Richard Seaver and Austryn Wainhouse. On Sade: Timo Airaksinen, *The Philosophy of the Marquis de Sade* (Routledge, 1995). On the Enlightenment in general, I was also guided by Anna Clark's *Desire: A History of Human Sexuality* (Routledge, 2008). David Hume's sketchy passages on the relationship between beauty, benevolence, and lust are in the second part of the second book of *A Treatise of Human Nature* (JM Dent and Sons, 1949), section XI.

On Kant: Alan Soble, 'Kant and Sexual Perversion', *The Monist* 86 1 (2003), 55–89; Irving Singer, 'The Morality of Sex: Contra Kant', *Critical Horizons* 1 2 (2000), 175–91. Ryan Patrick Hanley highlights the more egalitarian parts of Kant's ideas in 'Kant's Sexual Contract', *The Journal of Politics* 76 4 (2014), pp.914–27. Kant is also used to defend autonomy, though conflicts arise between his enlightenment values and his Christian conservatism: Thomas Mappes, 'Sexual Morality and the Concept of Using Another Person', Howard Klepper, 'Sexual Exploitation and the Value of Persons', and Alan Soble, 'Sexual Use', all of which are from *The Philosophy of Sex: Contemporary Readings* (Rowman and Littlefield, 2008), edited by Alan Soble and Nicholas Power. On Hegel: Edward C. Halper, 'Hegel's Family Values', *The Review of Metaphysics*, 54, 4 (2001), 815–58; Joan B. Landes, 'Hegel's Conception of the Family', *Polity* 14 1 (1981), 5–28; David West, *Reason and Sexuality in Western Thought* (Polity, 2005), 138–45.

Arthur Schopenhauer is never shy about sex, but his most thorough discussion is in 'Metaphysics of Sexual Love'. This is a supplement in *The World as Will and Representation*, Volume 2 (Cambridge University Press, 2018), edited and translated by Judith Norman, Alistair Welchman, and Christopher Janaway. It is also available in cheaper essay collections, and for free electronically in older translations.

For an excellent introduction to philosophy's man problem, see: Fiona Jenkins and Katrina Hutchinson's 'Searching For Sofia: Gender and Philosophy in the 21st Century', in *Women in Philosophy: What Needs to Change?* (Oxford, 2013), edited by Jenkins and Hutchinson. On why this matters: Marylin Friedman's 'Why Should We Care?', in the same volume. On possible causes and solutions: AE Kings, 'Understanding the Underrepresentation of Women and Minorities in Philosophy', *Metaphilosophy* 50 3 (2019), 212–30. On the need for new histories of philosophy, which show women's contributions *and* how these were denied: Sarah Hutton, 'Women, philosophy and the history of philosophy', *British Journal for the History of Philosophy* 27 4 (2019), 684–701. On gender and race in philosophy:

V. Denise James, 'A Black Feminist Philosopher: Is
That Possible?', *Hypatia* 29 1 (2014), 189–95; and
George Yancy, 'Situated Black Women's Voices in/on the
Profession of Philosophy', *Hypatia* 23 2 (2008), 155–9.
I am still thinking about Yancy's quote from philosopher
Anita Allen: 'Two very prominent philosophers offered
to look at my resume (I was flattered) and then asked to
sleep with me (I was disturbed).'

Speaking of terrible ideas about women: Friedrich
Nietzsche, *Ecce Homo* (Penguin, 1992), translated by
RJ Hollingdale. James Boswell's three columns titled
'On Love' are from *Boswell's Column* (William Kimber,
1951). He used the pseudonym 'The Hypochrondriack'.

On gratification: Roger Crisp and Morten Kringelbach,
'Higher and Lower Pleasures Revisited: Evidence from
Neuroscience', *Neuroethics* 11 2 (2018), 211–15.

Martha Nussbaum's *The Fragility of Goodness*
(Cambridge University Press, 1989) is an exceptional
work of modern Aristotelian scholarship, which refuses to
do 'neutral' philosophy. It is also a fine reading of Greek
tragedy, which dares to be moved — and to emphasise
that this movement is moral.

Virginia Woolf's essays remain a highpoint for the
form. And her essays on essays are especially good. Both
quoted here can be found in her *Selected Essays* (Oxford
University Press, 2008), edited by David Bradshaw.
I also have her four-volume collected essays, edited by
her husband Leonard (Chatto and Windus, 1969). But
they are missing 'The Decay of Essay-Writing', for some
reason. Jacques Barzun's 'Venus at Large' is in *Encounter*
26 (1966), 24–30. Sartre's quip on writing is from 'Why
Write?', in his *Literature and Existentialism* (Citadel
Press, 1962), translated by Bernard Frechtman. Audre

Lorde's 'The Uses of the Erotic' is from *Sister Outlaw* (Crossing Press, 2007). And Ann Patchett discusses the joy of sharing literature in 'Need a good book? Novelist Ann Patchett would like to tell you what to read', *The Washington Post* (April 27th, 2015).

John Dewey's *Art as Experience* (Minton, Balch and Company, 1934) remains a clear, enthusiastic and typically down-to-earth theory of art. 'The Sovereignty of Good Over Other Concepts', from *The Sovereignty of Good* (Routledge, 2007) is not exactly down-to-earth. This is the wrong metaphor. But it is yet another invitation away from selfishness and illusion. Stuart Hampshire, 'Philosophy and Fantasy', *The New York Review of Books* (September 26th, 1968).

A Warning

Kate Manne's discussion of trauma is in 'Why I Use Trigger Warnings', *The New York Times* (September 19th, 2015).

The Vulgar, Not the Vulgate

The discussion of Norman French's status is in Henry and Renée Kahane, 'Decline and Survival of Western Prestige Languages', *Language* 55 1 (1979), 183–98. Henry James's *The Portrait of Lady* is out of copyright, and available cheaply or for free. I have a nice blue hardback, published by Oxford University Press (1958), with an introduction by Graham Greene ('this master-craftsman always has his reasons'). HG Wells's *Love and Mrs*

Lewisham is also widely available. I read it here: http://www.gutenberg.org/files/11640/11640-h/11640-h.htm. All the etymology and historical examples are from the complete *Oxford English Dictionary*, which I accessed through my university. The handsome print edition runs to twenty volumes, and is quite expensive indeed.

Markus Gabriel's *Why the World Does Not Exist* (Polity, 2015) is a breathlessly clever discussion of our abstractions (including 'the world' as a totality).

Clowns

Alas, my paperback of Ian McEwan's *On Chesil Beach* (Vintage, 2018) is the movie edition. I owned the much-nicer hardback (Jonathan Cape, 2007), but gave it away as a gift.

Simone de Beauvoir's *The Second Sex* (Penguin, 1972) is translated by HM Parshley. An enormous and enormously powerful work of feminist philosophy. My copy is falling to pieces — from enthusiasm, not neglect.

The ancient Greek conversation about boners is from Aristophanes, *Birds, Lysistrata, Women at the Thesmophoria* (Loeb Classical Library, 2000), edited and translated by Jeffrey Henderson. Montaigne's discussion of the same is from 'On the power of the imagination', from *The Complete Essays* (Penguin, 2004), translated by MA Screech.

Marilyn French, *The Women's Room* (Hachette, 1993). Krissy Kneen's tentacular 'The Dream of the Fisherman's Wife' is in *Triptych* (Text, 2011), along with 'Susanna' and 'Romulus and Remus'. John Bromyard's slur is from his fourteenth-century *Summa Predicantium* entry on beauty, and quoted by Susan Haskins in *Mary Magdalen: Truth and Myth* (Pimlico, 2005), 153. Jeanette Winterson's typically sensuous phrase is from her *Written on the Body* (Vintage, 2014). For shameless horny fun, Linda Jaivin's 'The Road to Gundagai' and other stories are collected in *Eat Me* (Text, 1995).

For shameless horny fun, do not read Martin Heidegger's *Being and Time* (Basil Blackwell, 1973), translated by John Macquarrie and Edward Robinson. Let me be clear: Heidegger was an antisemitic prick, and his legacy is ethically marred. But his ideas helped to shape mine, and it would be false to deny this.

Carmen Maria Machado's 'Inventory' is from *Her Body and Other Parties* (Serpent's Tail, 2018). Visceral, sometimes hallucinatory fiction — and written with nuance and force.

Michael Clarke, 'Humour and Incongruity', *Philosophy* 45 171 (1970), 20–32. See also Bob Plant, 'Absurdity, Incongruity and Laughter', *Philosophy* 84 (2009), 111–34.

Samuel Johnson's quip is from *The Rambler* 194 (January 25th, 1752). But I first read it in the mouth of Doctor Stephen Maturin in one of Patrick O'Brian's brilliant naval adventures, *Post Captain* (HarperCollins, 2016). Henri Bergson, *Laughter: An Essay on the Meaning of the Comic* (Dover, 2005), translated by Cloudesley Brereton and Fred Rothwell. Noël Carroll, 'Horror and Humor', *The Journal of Aesthetics and Art Criticism* 57 2 (1999), 145–60. Thomas Nagel, 'The Absurd', in *Mortal Questions* (Cambridge University Press, 2013).

Friedrich Nietzsche's *The Gay Science* (Vintage, 1974) is not nearly as queer as it might sound, but it is a joyous 'yes' to existence. My paperback is translated by Walter Kaufman, but others are available easily and cheaply. Thomas Hobbes, *Leviathan* (Everyman, 1973). Ralph Waldo Emerson's 'Circles' is from *Selected Essays* (Penguin, 1982), but available electronically for free.

The John Ruskin observation about penguins is from his letter to Charles Eliot Norton, November 4th 1860. From *The Letters of John Ruskin to Charles Eliot Norton* (Houghton, Mifflin and Company, 1904). Milan Kundera, *The Unbearable Lightness of Being* (Faber and Faber, 1999), translated by Michael Henry Heim.

Less about gymnastic screwing and more about elite male sexuality: Vatsyayana's *Kama Sutra: A Guide to the Art of Pleasure* (Penguin, 2012), translated by AND Haksar. Sharyn Graham Davis, 'The transcendent bissu', *Aeon*, available here: https://aeon.co/essays/the-west-can-learn-from-southeast-asias-transgender-heritage. Matthew Looper, 'Women-Men (and Men-Women): Classic Maya Rulers and the Third Gender', in *Ancient Maya Women* (AltaMira Press, 2002), edited by Traci Arden. See also Miranda K. Stockett, 'On the importance of difference: re-envisioning sex and gender in ancient Mesoamerica', *World Archaeology* 37 4 (2005), 566–78. On the 'third gender' in South Asia: Walter Penrose, 'Hidden in History: Female Homoeroticism and Women of a "Third Nature" in the South Asian Past', *Journal of the History of Sexuality* 10 1 (2001), 3–39. Robin Dembroff, 'Why be nonbinary?', *Aeon*: https://aeon.co/essays/nonbinary-identity-is-a-radical-stance-against-gender-segregation.

Jeremy Hua, Kerry Hildreth and Victoria Pelak, 'Effects of Testosterone Therapy on Cognitive Function in Aging: A Systematic Review', *Cognitive and Behavioral Neurology* 29 3 (2016), 122–38. Robert Martin, *How We Do It* (Basic Books, 2013).

Virginia Woolf, *Orlando* (Alma Classics, 2014). I bought myself a fancy hardcover edition because I am fancy, but this is everywhere — cheap or free.

Aristotle discusses 'ready-wittedness' in his *Nicomachean Ethics*, translated by WD Ross, in *The Complete Works of Aristotle* (Princeton University Press, 1991), edited by Jonathan Barnes. Thucydides, *History of the Peloponnesian War*, Volume I (Loeb Classical Library, 1919), translated by CF Smith. On *eutrapelia*: Pat Arneson, 'Playful Seriousness: The Virtue of Eutrapelia in Dialogue', *Dialogue* 26 1 (2018), 46–58. Also see: John Lippit, 'Is a Sense of Humour a Virtue', *The Monist* 88 1 (2005), 72–92.

John Updike, 'Elderly Sex', in *John Updike: Selected Poems* (Alfred A Knopf, 2015), edited by Christopher Cardiff. Ellen Bass's marvellous 'The Morning After' is from *Like a Beggar* (Copper Canyon Press, 2014). Alain Badiou, *In Praise of Love* (Serpent's Tale, 2012), translated by Peter Bush.

Bubbles

I did not expect to find myself eagerly seeking out foreskin research, but curiosity is curiosity: Johann Friedrich Meckel, *Manual of Descriptive and Pathological Anatomy* (E Henderson, 1838), translated from the German by Antoine Jacques Louis Jourdan and Gilbert Breschet, and from the French into English by AS Doane. Joseph Hyrtl, 'Practical Remarks on the Surgical Anatomy of the Penis' (1847), translated by JC M'Mechan, *The Medical and Surgical Reporter* XXXII (1875). On Hyrtl's vitalism, see: Gerald Wiest and Robert Baloh, 'The Personal and

Scientific Feud Between Ernst Brücke and Josef Hyrtl', *Otology and Neurotology* 27 (2006), 570–75. Luciano Alves Favorito, Carlos Miguel Balassiano, Waldemar Silva Costa and Francisco José Barcellos Sampaio, 'Development of the human foreskin during the fetal period', *Histology & Histopathology* 27 8 (2012), 1041–5. Ken McGrath, 'The Frenular Delta: a New Preputial Structure', in *Understanding Circumcision* (Springer, 2001), edited by CG Denniston, FM Hodges, and MF Milos. See also Brian Earp, 'Infant circumcision and adult penile sensitivity: implications for sexual experience', *Trends in Urology and Men's Health* (July/August 2016).

Roland Barthes's *The Lover's Discourse* (Vintage, 2002), translated by Richard Howard, is a hugely suggestive meditation on romance. For me, it highlights the psychological work of love: the way we labour to maintain a very peculiar state of mind. Carol Ann Duffy, 'Warming Her Pearls' from *Selling Manhattan* (Anvil Press, 1987). Ovid, *Metamorphoses* (Penguin, 1955), translated by Mary Innes.

On human time: Edmund Husserl, *Phenomenology of Internal Time-Consciousness* (Indiana University Press, 1964), translated by James Churchill; David Carr, *Time, Narrative, and History* (Indiana University Press, 1986); David Herman and Becky Childs, 'Narrative and Cognition in Beowulf', *Style* 37 2 (2003), 177–202.

My own brief discussion of reading less (all evidence to the contrary) is the chapter 'Temperance', from *The Art of Reading* (Scribe, 2018). Alasdair MacIntyre's *After Virtue* (Duckworth, 1984) remains *the* modern conservative defence of virtue theory. Alessandro Baricco, *Silk* (Text, 2006), translated by Ann Golstein. *The Arabian Nights: Tales of 1001 Nights*, Volume 1 (Penguin,

2010), translated by Malcolm Lyons with Ursula Lyons. Michael Austin, 'The Influence of Anxiety and Literature's Panglossian Nose', *Philosophy and Literature* 31 (2007), 215–32.

Erving Goffman's *Encounters* (Penguin, 1961) is sociology at its most lucid and conversational.

Nagata Kabi, *My Lesbian Experience With Loneliness* (Seven Seas, 2017), translated by Jocelyne Allen.

Pedro J. Nobre and Jose Pinto-Gouveia, 'Emotions During Sexual Activity: Differences Between Sexually Functional and Dysfunctional Men and Women', *Archives of Sexual Behaviour* 35 (2006), 491–99.

On transgender sexuality: J Hess, A Henkel, J Bohr, C Rehme, A Panic, L Panic, R Rossi Neto, B Hadaschik, Y Hess, 'Sexuality after Male-to-Female Gender Affirmation Surgery', *Biomed Research International* (May 27th 2018); Sanne Nikkelen and Baudewijntje Kreukels, 'Sexual Experiences in Transgender People: The Role of Desire for Gender-Conforming Interventions, Psychological Well-being, and Body Satisfaction', *Journal of Sex and Marital Therapy* 44 4 (2018), 370–81; Shoshana Rosenberg, PJ Matt Tilley, Julia Morgan, '"I Couldn't Imagine My Life Without It": Australian TransWomen's Experiences of Sexuality, Intimacy, and Gender-Affirming Hormone Therapy', *Sexuality and Culture* 23 (2019), 962–77.

Though many decades old, this analysis of gendered value is still frustratingly relevant: Anne Phillips and Barbara Taylor, 'Sex and Skill: Notes Towards a Feminist Economics', *Feminist Review* 6 1 (1980), 79–88.

My favourite novel, from one of my favourite authors: Virginia Woolf, *Mrs Dalloway* (Oxford University Press, 2000). SA Jones's *The Fortress* (Echo, 2018) is a confronting but also very sexy feminist work.

Brooke Magnanti's quip is from her *The Intimate Adventures of a London Call Girl* (Weidenfeld & Nicolson, 2010) writing as Belle de Jour.

Tiresias' Secret

I typically prefer Robert Fagles' modern translation of Homer's *Iliad*, which I have in a handsome Folio Society edition (1997). But I do like the rhyming verve of Pope's interpretation, in *The Iliad and Odyssey of Homer* (George Routledge and Sons, 1884), and available electronically for free. Zeus's smug reply to Hera is from Ovid's *Metamorphoses*. Robert Graves, *The Greek Myths*, published by the Folio Society (2001).

Jordy Rosenberg's *Confessions of the Fox* (Atlantic, 2018) has plenty of suggestive screwing, but also equally suggestive screwing with history and power. Clever, thrilling, moving.

The warning about goddesses is from Homer's hymn to Aphrodite, in *Homeric Hymns, Homeric Apocrypha, Lives of Homer* (Loeb Classical Library, 2003), translated by Martin West.

Ocean Vuong's *On Earth We're Briefly Gorgeous* (Jonathan Cape, 2019) is a masterful portrait of trauma and love.

Wendy Heywood and Anthony Smith, 'Anal sex practices in heterosexual and male homosexual populations: A review of population-based data', *Sexual Health* 9 6 (2012), 512–26. Stephen Fry, *Moab is my Washpot* (Arrow, 2004).

Sara Johnsdotter, 'Discourses on sexual pleasure after genital modifications: the fallacy of genital determinism (a response to J. Steven Svoboda)', *Global Discourse* 3 2 (2013), 256–65.

Thomas Nagel's famous 'bat' essay is from *Mortal Questions*. John Money's almost-as-famous description of orgasm has a more complicated provenance. Joann Ellison Rodgers quotes him in *Sex: A Natural History* (Times Books, 2001), but the original text is not specified. I asked Rodgers about this, but she was not sure of the exact source. I trust her scholarship.

Georges Bataille, *Eroticism: Death and Sensuality* (City Lights Books, 1986), translated by Mary Dalwood. Bataille is very interesting and often quite challenging — until he gets to gender. How very philosophical of him.

On facial ejaculation, tasting cum, and genitals: Carina Hsieh, '3 Women Get Brutally Honest About Why They Love or Hate Facials', *Cosmopolitan* (April 14th 2017); Anaïs Nin, *Henry and June* (Penguin, 2001); Sharon Olds, 'The Connoisseuse of Slugs', *The Dead and the Living* (Alfred Knopf, 1984); Rita Dove, 'After Reading *Mickey in the Night Kitchen* for the Third Time Before Bed', *Collected Poems: 1974–2004* (WW Norton, 2017).

Ludwig Wittgenstein, *Philosophical Investigations* (Basil Blackwell, 1991), translated by GEM Anscombe.

Apollodorus, *The Library of Greek Mythology* (Oxford University Press, 1997), translated by Robin Hard.

Choke Me

Clive Barker, *Imajica* (Harper Collins, 1991). Identifying what is formative can be an exercise in retrospective mythology, but I do reckon Barker's transgressive genders and sexualities helped to loosen my youthful categories.

Richard von Krafft-Ebing, *Psychopathia Sexualis* (The FA Davis Company, 1894), translated by Charles Gilbert Chaddock.

On the frequency of so-called 'rape fantasies': Joseph Critelli and Jenny Bivona, 'Women's erotic rape fantasies: an evaluation of theory and research', *Journal of Sex Research* 45 1 (2008), 57–70; Christian Joyal and Julie Carpentier, 'The Prevalence of Paraphilic Interests and Behaviors in the General Population: A Provincial Survey', *Journal of Sex Research* 54 2 (2017), 161–71.

John Norman's *Vagabonds of Gor* (James Bennett, 1987). The novels prompted a 'Gorean' subculture of domination and submission play. On this, see: Jeremy Wilson, 'Behind Gor, a "slave master" subculture of sexual deviance', *Daily Dot* (March 31st, 2014), available here: https://www.dailydot.com/irl/gor-gorean-slaves-history/.

Sally Rooney's *Normal People* (Faber and Faber, 2018) is a finely observed study of romance, psychology, and class in modern Ireland.

On BDSM: Shannon Martin, Felix Smith, and Stuart Quirk, 'Discriminating Coercive from Sadomasochistic Sexuality', *Archives of Sexual Research* 45 5 (2015); Pamela Connolly, 'Psychological Functioning of Bondage/ Domination/Sado-Masochism (BDSM) Practitioners', *Journal of Psychology & Human Sexuality* 18 1 (2006), 79–120; Sallie Tisdale, 'Talk Dirty to Me', in *The Philosophy of Sex: Contemporary Readings*; Corie Hammers, 'Reworking Trauma through BDSM', *Signs* 2 (2019), 491–514.

On hypoxyphilia and such: Torsten Passie, Uew Hartmann, Udo Schneider, Hinderk Emrich, 'On the function of groaning and hyperventilation during sexual intercourse: intensification of sexual experience by altering brain metabolism through hypocapnia', *Medican Hypotheses* 60 5 (2003), 660–63; Stephen Hucker, 'Hypoxyphilia', *Archives of Sexual Behavior* 40 6 (2011), 1323–26.

Science on depression, anxiety, and lust: Sean Laurent and Anne Simons, 'Sexual dysfunction in depression and anxiety: Conceptualising sexual dysfunction as part of an internalising dimension', *Clinical Psychological Review* 29 (2009), 573–85; Tera Beaber and Paul Werner, 'The Relationship Between Anxiety and Sexual Functioning in Lesbians and Heterosexual Women', *Journal of Homosexuality* 56 (2009), 639–54; Andrea Bradford and Cindy Meston, 'The impact of anxiety on sexual arousal in women', *Behaviour Research and Therapy* 44 (2006), 1067–77; BB de Lucena and CHN Abdo, 'Personal factors that contribute to or impair women's ability to achieve orgasm', *International Journal of Impotence Research* 26 5 (2014), 177–81.

Literature on depression, anxiety, and lust: F Scott Fitzgerald, 'The Crack-Up', in *The Crack-Up With Other Pieces and Stories* (Penguin, 1974); Roxane Gay's 'Bone Density', in *Difficult Women* (Corsair, 2017); David Cronenberg, *Consumed* (4th Estate, 2014); Anaïs Nin, 'The Woman on the Dunes', *Little Birds* (Penguin, 2002).

Embodiment and BDSM: Siyang Luo and Xiao Zhang, 'Embodiment and Humiliation Moderation of Neural Responses to Others' Suffering in Female Submissive BDSM Practitioners', *Frontiers in Neuroscience* 12 463 (2018); Siyang Luo and Xiao Zhang, 'Empathy in female submissive BDSM practitioners', *Neuropsychologia* 116 (2018), 44–51.

Embodiment more generally: Friedrich Nietzsche, 'Of the Despisers of the Body' in *Thus Spoke Zarathustra* (Penguin, 1969), translated by RJ Hollingdale; Merleau-Ponty's *The Phenomenology of Perception*; George Lakoff and Mark Johnson, *Metaphors We Live By* (University of Chicago Press, 1981).

Edmund White, *States of Desire* (Picador, 1986).

On 'druthers', see Robin Dembroff, 'What is Sexual Orientation?', *Philosopher's Imprint* 16 3 (2016), 1–27. On berserkers, see Michael Speidel, 'Berserks: A History of Indo-European "Mad Warriors", *Journal of World History* 13 2 (2002), 253–90.

DH Lawrence, *The White Peacock* (Penguin, 1995). Catherine Robbe-Grillet is quoted by Nicole Disser, in '85-year-old French Dominatrix and Her Concubine Let Us Into Their Chateau of Cruelty', *Bedford+Bowery*, available here: https://bedfordandbowery.com/2015/ 10/85-year-old-dominatrix-and-her-concubine-let-us-into-their-chateau-of-cruelty/. Timo Airaksinen, 'A philosophical and rhetorical theory of BDSM', *The Journal of Mind and Behavior* 38 1 (2017), 53–73.

Solomon Kane's Demon

Solomon Kane is a weird guy, but he is very much a *guy*. And his mythos is telling. 'The Cold Hands of Death', written by Don Glut and illustrated by Steve Gan and Dino Castrillo, in *The Saga of Solomon Kane*, edited by Katie Moody (Dark Horse Books, 2009). All of Robert E. Howard's original Kane stories are collected in *The Savage Tales of Solomon Kane* (Del Rey, 1998), edited by Rusty Burke.

On the succubus: *Isaiah* 34:14, here in the King James translation; Grover Sandeep, Mehra Aseem, Dua Devakshi, 'Unusual cases of succubus: A cultural phenomenon manifesting as part of psychopathology', *Industrial Psychiatry Journal* 27 1 (2018), 147–50; Ann Cox, 'Sleep paralysis and folklore', *Clinical Review* 6 7 (2015), 1–4; *The Zohar* (The Soncino Press, 1984), translated by Harry Sperling and Maurice Simon.

On the *ezigbo mmada*: Christopher Agulanna, 'Ezigbo Mmadu: An Exploration of the Igbo Concept of a Good Person', *The Journal of Pan African Studies* 4 5 (2011), 139–61; Chinyere Ukpokolo, 'Ezigbo Mmadu: An Anthropological Investigation Into the Concept of a Good Person in Igbo Worldview', *Prajñā Vihāra* 12 1 (2011), 29–44.

On African aesthetics: Justin Njiofor, 'The Concept of Beauty: A Study in African Aesthetics', *Asian Journal of Social Sciences & Humanities* 7 3 (2018), 30–40; Rowland Abiodun, 'African Aesthetics', The Journal of Aesthetic Education 35 4 (2001), 15–23; Diana-Abasi Ibanga, 'The Concept of Beauty in African Philosophy', *Africology: The Journal of Pan African Studies* 10 7 (2017), 249–60.

The madness of love is supposedly everywhere, but my references here are: Anne Carson, *Eros the Bittersweet* (Dalkey Archive Press, 2005); Thomas Moore's 'The Time I've Lost in Wooing', https://www.poetryfoundation.org/poems/44783/the-time-ive-lost-in-wooing; Shakespeare's Sonnet 147, from *Shakespeare's Sonnets* (Penguin, 2009); Petrarch, Sonnet 141, in *Petrarch: The Canzoniere, or Rerum Vulgarium Fragmenta* (Indiana University Press, 1999), translated by Mark Musa.

Leonard Woolf's *Sowing* (The Hogarth Press, 1961)

is part of a five-volume autobiography, which gives an extraordinarily rich portrait of Woolf's life and times (including his years in colonial Sri Lanka), and marriage to Virginia. John Clare's 'First Love' is from *John Clare: Selected Works* (Oxford University Press, 2008), edited by Eric Robinson and David Powell.

Research on beauty: Vicki Ritts, Miles Patterson, Mark Tubbs, 'Expectations, Impressions, and Judgments of Physically Attractive Students: A Review', *Review of Educational Research* 62 4 (1992), pp. 413–426; Sean Talamas, Kenneth Mavor, David Perrett, 'Blinded by Beauty: Attractiveness Bias and Accurate Perceptions of Academic Performance', *PLoS ONE* 11 2 (2016), 1–18; Emanuela Sala, Marco Terraneo, Mario Lucchini, Gundi Knies, 'Exploring the impact of male and female facial attractiveness on occupational prestige', *Research in Social Stratification and Mobility* 31 (2013), 69–81; Megumi Hosodo, Eugene Stone-Romero, Gwen Coats, 'The Effects of Physical Attractiveness on Job-Related Outcomes: A Meta-Analysis of Experimental Studies', *Personnel Psychology* 56 (2003), 431–62.

I was introduced to Bourdieu's work as an undergraduate, and his work remains relevant. Pierre Bourdieu and Loïc Wacquant, *An Invitation to Reflexive Sociology* (1992); Pierre Bourdieu, *The Logic of Practice* (Polity Press, 1992), translated by Richard Nice. See also: Kathleen O'Connor and Eric Gladstone, 'Beauty and social capital: Being attractive shapes social networks', *Social Networks* 52 (2018), 42–7; Catherine Hakim, 'Erotic Capital', *European Sociological Review* 26 5 (2010), 499–518.

Suppose we ask the Other? Here is a start: Gabriel García Márquez, 'Eva is Inside Her Cat', in *Innocent*

Eréndira and Other Stories (Penguin, 2014), translated by Gregory Rabassa; Lucia Berlin, 'Sex Appeal', from *A Manual for Cleaning Women* (Picador, 2015), edited by Stephen Emerson; Jennifer Clement, *Prayers for the Stolen* (Vintage, 2014); AS Byatt, 'The Djinn in the Nightingale's Eye', in *The Djinn in the Nightingale's Eye: Five Fairy Stories* (Vintage, 1995); Pat Barker, *The Silence of the Girls* (Hamish Hamilton, 2018).

On racist Robert E Howard and his racist buddy HP Lovecraft, see my 'Aryans in Love', *Meanjin* 79 2 (2020). Chinua Achebe, 'An Image of Africa: Racism in Conrad's Heart of Darkness', *The Massachusetts Review* 57 1 (2016), 14–27. Danice Brown, Rhonda White-Johnson, Felicia Griffin-Fennell, 'Breaking the chains: examining the endorsement of modern Jezebel images and racial-ethnic esteem among African American women', *Culture, Health & Sexuality* 15 5 (2013), 525–39.

Friedrich Nietzsche, *Twilight of the Idols/The Anti-Christ* (Penguin, 1990), translated by RJ Hollingdale. By the same author, *The Birth of Tragedy* (Penguin, 1993) is translated by Shaun Whiteside. Thomas Mann, *Death in Venice, Tristan, Tonio Kröger* (Penguin, 1983), translated by HT Lowe-Porter.

The Face of Nakedness

John Banville, *The Infinities* (Picador, 2009).

For an overview of the evolutionary value of beauty, see the third chapter of Joann Ellison Rogers's *Sex: A Natural History*. For a more recent discussion of the literature, especially the observable but small effects of symmetry on female faces: Alex Jones and Bastian

Jaeger, 'Biological Bases of Beauty Revisited: The Effect of Symmetry, Averageness, and Sexual Dimorphism on Female Facial Attractiveness', *Symmetry* 11 2 (2019). On the subjective contribution to judgements of facial beauty: Johannes Hönekopp, 'Once More: Is Beauty in the Eye of the Beholder? Relative Contributions of Private and Shared Taste to Judgments of Facial Attractiveness', *Journal of Experimental Psychology* 32 2 (2006), 199–209. More generally, on the perceiver's role in perception: Eric Hehman, Clare Sutherland, Jessica Flake, and Michael Slepian, 'The Unique Contributions of Perceiver and Target Characteristics in Person Perception', *Journal of Personality and Social Psychology* 113 4 (2017), 513–29.

George Santayana, *The Sense of Beauty* (The Modern Library, 1955). Ruth Barcan, *Nudity: A Cultural Anatomy* (Bloomsbury, 2004). Homer's *Odyssey*, from *The Iliad and Odyssey of Homer*.

Hans Jonas, 'The Nobility of Sight', *Philosophy and Phenomenological Research* 14 4 (1954), 507–19. John Dewey, *Reconstruction in Philosophy* (University of London Press, 1921).

Examples of nudity in other senses: Angela Carter, 'The Tiger's Bride', in *The Bloody Chamber and Other Stories* (Vintage, 2006); Sarah Perry, *The Essex Serpent* (Serpent's Tail, 2016); Deborah Levy, 'Vienna', in *Black Vodka* (And Other Stories, 2013).

Calvin's ideas about nudity are discussed in Nora Martin Peterson's 'The Impossible Striptease: Nudity in Jean Calvin and Michel de Montaigne', *Renaissance and Reformation* 37 1 (2014), 65–85. Moyo Okediji looks into nudity for the Yoruba in 'The Naked Truth: Nude Figures in Yoruba Art', *Journal of Black Studies* 22 1 (1991), 30–44.

Roland Barthes, 'Striptease', in *Mythologies* (Vintage, 2009), translated by Annette Lavers. Barthes' 'The Face of Garbo' is from the same collection. James Arieti, 'Nudity in Greek Athletics', *The Classical World* 68 7 (1975), 431–6.

Milan Kundera's 'The Hitchhiking Game' is from *Laughable Loves* (Faber and Faber, 1991), translated by Suzanne Rappaport. My *Mahābhārata* (Penguin, 2009) is translated by John D Smith.

Irenäus Eibl-Eibesfeldt, *Love and Hate: On the natural history of basic behaviour patterns* (Methuen and Co., 1971), Geoffrey Strachan.

Christopher Marlowe's *Doctor Faustus* from *Faustus and Other Plays* (Oxford University Press, 2008).

Alone with Enki

On Enki, Atum, and Prajapati, I was guided by references in David Leeming's *Sex in the World of Myth* (Reaction Books, 2018) — though not always by his interpretations. The passages on Enki are from the Electronic Corpus of Sumerian Literature, provided by the Faculty of Oriental Studies, University of Oxford. Available here: http://etcsl. orinst.ox.ac.uk/. On Enki, see also: Keith Dickson, 'Enki and Ninhursag: The Trickster in Paradise', *Journal of Near Eastern Studies* 66 1 (2007), 1–32; Hannes Galter, 'The Mesopotamian God Enki/Ea', *Religion Compass* 9 3 (2015), 66–76. On Heliopolis and Atum: Nuzzolo Massimiliano and Krejčí Jaromír, 'Heliopolis and the Solar Cult in the Third Millennium BC', *Egypt and the Levant* 27 (2017), 357–79. Julius Eggeling's translation of the Satapatha Brahmana can be found in *Readings in Eastern Religions* (Wilfrid Laurier University Press, 2007), edited by Harold Coward, Ronald Neufeldt, Eva K. Neumaier. It is also available electronically.

Various creation myths are detailed in David Leeming's *The Oxford Companion to World Mythology* (Oxford University Press, 2005). Ymir's bloody end is from *The Poetic Edda* (Oxford University Press, 1999), translated by Carolyne Larrington. Hesiod's *Theogony* is from *Hesiod and Theognis* (Penguin, 1973), translated by Dorothea Wender. On the Shabaka Stone and Memphis theology: Joshua Bodine, 'The Shabaka Stone: An Introduction', *Studia Antiqua* 7 1 (2009), 1–21.

Roberto Calasso's arboreal metaphor comes from his interview with Lila Azam Zanganeh in *The Paris Review* 202 (2012). Nietzsche's tirade against the Church is from *The Anti-Christ*. James Brundage's summary of Christian 'tension' is from the introduction to his *Law, Sex, and Christian Society in Medieval Europe* (University of Chicago Press, 1987). Jerome's warning: Jerome, *Against Jovinianus* (Dalcassian Publishing, 2017), translated by WH Fremantle. Kathy Gaca, *The Making of Fornication: Eros, Ethics, and Political Reform in Greek Philosophy and Early Christianity* (University of California Press, 2017).

Roy Levin's good news for wankers: 'Sexual activity, health and well-being — the beneficial roles of coitus and masturbation', *Sexual and Relationship Therapy* 22 1 (2007), 135–48. Eli Coleman's discussion of jerking off and autonomy is from 'Masturbation as a Means of Achieving Sexual Health', *Journal of Psychology & Human Sexuality* 14 2/3 (2002), 5–16. See also William Phipps's historical and medical overview in 'Masturbation: Vice or Virtue?', *Journal of Religion and Health* 16 3 (1977), 183–95.

Michel Foucault's discussion of 'intervening' is from 'The Minimalist Self', in *Politics, Philosophy, Culture: Interviews and Other Writings 1977–84* (Routledge, 1990), edited by Lawrence Kritzman.

When I was a child, I thought James Joyce's *Ulysses* was about an archer not a wanker: there was a Greek bow on the cover of my father's edition. My Bodley Head (1976) edition is less fancy, but is still holding together after four decades.

Immanuel Kant, *The Doctrine of Virtue* (University of Pennsylvania Press, 1964), translated by Mary Gregor. On rates of masturbation and fantasy by gender, see Harold Leitenberg and Kris Henning's review of the literature: 'Sexual Fantasy', *Psychological Bulletin* 117 3 (1995), 469–96. On asexuals: Morag Yule, Lori Brotto, Boris Gorzalka, 'Sexual fantasy and masturbation among asexual individuals', *The Canadian Journal of Human Sexuality* 23 2 (2014), 89–95.

Clement's *Exhortation to the Heathen* is from *The Ante-Nicene Fathers: Volume II* (T & T Clark, 1867–73), translated and edited by Alexander Roberts and James Donaldson. Mircea Eliade's observation is from *Myths, Rites, Symbols*, Volume 2 (Harper and Row, 1976), edited by Wendell Beane and William Doty.

On masturbation in other animals: Daniel Engber, 'Hands or Paws or Anything They Got', *Slate* (July 16th, 2009), available here: https://slate.com/technology/2009/07/do-animals-masturbate.html. Immanuel Kant said 'no' to jerking off but 'yes' to labour in his *Lectures on Ethics* (Harper Torchbooks, 1963), translated by Louis Infield. Kant and masturbation are discussed by Soble and Singer. On wanking as a problem for the eighteenth-century middle classes: Michael

Stolberg, 'An Unmanly Vice: Self-Pollution, Anxiety, and the Body in the Eighteenth Century', *The Social History of Medicine* 13 1 (2000), 1–21; Franz Eder, 'Discourse and Sexual Desire: German-Language Discourse on Masturbation in the Late Eighteenth Century', *Journal of the History of Sexuality* 13 4 (2004), 428–45.

CS Lewis's warning about jerking off is from a letter to Keith Masson in *The Collected Letters of C. S. Lewis*, Volume III (HarperOne, 2007), edited by Walter Hooper. Alan Soble's 'Masturbation, Again' is from *The Philosophy of Sex: Contemporary Readings*. Arran Gare's *Nihilism Inc* (Eco-Logical Press, 1996) is, among other things, a study of European civilisation and its most cataclysmic tendencies. Frighteningly prescient.

Ibi Kaslik, *Skinny* (Bloomsbury, 2007). Samantha Allen, 'How I learned to orgasm after sex reassignment surgery', *Splinter* (25th October, 2016), available here: https://splinternews.com/how-i-learned-to-orgasm-after-sex-reassignment-surgery-1793863166. Ana Valens, 'Masturbation is tough for trans women. I know first-hand', *Daily Dot* (25th February, 2019): https://www.dailydot.com/irl/trans-sex-masturbation/.

Thomas Laqueur discusses female 'semen' and therapeutic masturbation in *Solitary Sex: A Cultural History of Masturbation* (Zone Books, 2003). Theodore's penitentials can be found in their original Anglo-Saxon and English here: http://www.anglo-saxon.net/penance/.

Adam Roberts, *Swiftly* (Gollancz, 2008); Alice Walker, *The Color Purple* (Weidenfeld & Nicolson, 2017).

Alfred Jules Ayer, *Language, Truth, and Logic* (Pelican, 1983).

Fuckzilla

The spuriously titled video is 'Kleio Gets Best Fuck of Her Life', starring Kleio Valentien and the Intruder. Available here: https://www.pornhub.com/view_video. php?viewkey=ph57cf38c4c6c59. I contacted the production company, actress and distributor for more information, but received no reply.

When Nietzsche lamented the humiliation of fine souls by Christianity, he was thinking of people like Blaise Pascal. Pascal's *Pensées* (Penguin, 1968) is translated by AJ Krailsheimer.

On men's sensitivity to their own erections: Meredith Chivers, Michael Seto, Martin Lalumière, Ellen Laan and Teresa Grimbos, 'Agreement of Self-Reported and Genital Measures of Sexual Arousal in Men and Women: A Meta-Analysis', *Archives of Sexual Behavior* 39 1 (2010), 5–56.

John Stoltenberg, 'How Men Have (a) Sex', *Refusing to be a Man: Essays on Social Justice* (Routledge, 2005).

Hannah Arendt's *The Human Condition* (Doubleday Anchor, 1958) is a proud and rightful defence of politics; of our power to communally build our common life, rather than just labouring or working. Roberto Calasso, *The Marriage of Cadmus and Harmony* (Vintage, 1994), translated by Tim Parks. I have quoted this brilliant study of myths and the mythic in all of my non-fiction books, and anyone who has read it ought to understand why.

Karel Čapek, *RUR* (Hachette, 2013), translated by Paul Selver and Nigel Playfair. Aeschylus' *Prometheus*, in *Prometheus Bound and Other Plays* (Penguin, 1961), translated by Philip Vellacott. Sarah Waters, *Tipping the Velvet* (Virago, 2011).

Alfred North Whitehead's suggestion that the universe might have been (or might be) otherwise is from *Dialogues of Alfred North Whitehead* XLIII (Max Reinhardt, 1954), as recorded by Lucien Price.

Shastra Deo's 'Chine' is from her collection *The Agonist* (University of Queensland Press, 2017), which includes some stunning meditations on the body, language, and passion.

Solidarity

In this chapter, the only quotes are from sex workers. I cite other sources, but do not quote them. I am not naive enough to believe this allows readers to hear some pure truths, without my noise. The idea is just to amplify voices that are typically silenced or shouted over.

On anal play, see Jonathan Branfman, Susan Stiritz, and Eric Anderson. 'Relaxing the Straight Male Anus: Decreasing Homohysteria around Anal Eroticism', *Sexualities* 21 1–2 (2018), 109–27.

Samuel Johnson's pompous lamentation is from *The Rambler* (5th November, 1751), and is given in the voice of a prostitute, Misella. Many of his works are available electronically, though they can be found together with introductory essays and notes here: *Selected Essays* (Penguin, 2003), edited by David Womersley. In the *Oxford English Dictionary*, 'prostitute' alone has various references from the sixteenth to the twentieth centuries. Many keep the Platonic metaphors of good and bad: above and below, lightness and heaviness, clean and dirty. This is without discussing 'whore', 'slut', and so on.

The Molnár quip is from *The Intimate Notebooks of George Jean Nathan* (1932, Alfred A Knopf), by George Jean Nathan. John Dryden's translation of Persius is *The satires of Decimus Junius Juvenalis translated into English verse by Mr. Dryden and several other eminent hands; together with the satires of Aulus Persius Flaccus, made English by Mr. Dryden; with explanatory notes at the end of each satire; to which is prefix'd a discourse concerning the original and progress of satire* (Jacob Tonson, 1693). Also available here: https://quod.lib.umich.edu/e/eebo/ A46439.0001.001?view=toc. Wolfgang Musculus's discussion of churches is from his *Common Places of Christian Religion* (R Wolfe, 1563), translated by John Man. *Polydore Vergil's English History*, Volume 1 (The Camden Society, 1846) was later edited by Henry Ellis. The discussion of Aethelred (called Etheldredus here) is from I.vii.255.

Veronica Monet on 'whore' is from 'Nothing But a Whore', available here: https://veronicamonet. wordpress.com/2008/01/06/nothing-but-a-whore/. The proportion of female sex workers is given by Fondation Scelles in *Current Assessment of the State of Prostitution* (2011): https://www.fondationscelles.org/ pdf/current-assessment-of-the-state-of-prostitution-2013. pdf, and reported widely. These figures might not be wholly reliable, as the work is often stigmatised and criminalised. On this, see: J Vandepitte, R Lyerla, G Dallabetta, F Crabbé, M Alary, A Buvé, 'Estimates of the number of female sex workers in different regions of the world', *Sexually Transmitted Infections* 82 Supplement 3 (2006), 18–25.

There has typically been less research on buyers than sellers of sex, though this has changed in recent years.

See Martin Monto, 'Female Prostitution, Customers, and Violence', *Violence Against Women* 10 2 (2004), 160–88. On the proportion of sex clients who are male rather than female, several reports and articles had no evidence for their claims, or cited research that had no evidence for their claims. In Australia, where sex work is legal, johns certainly are in the majority, janes in the minority: *Brothel Keeping and Sex Worker Services industry trends* (2014–2019), IBISWorld. For a more qualitative discussion of women buying sex: https://www.abc.net.au/news/2019–10–09/sex-industry-increase-in-australian-women-who-buy-sex/11578722.

Sarah Ditum on 'sex work': 'Why we shouldn't rebrand prostitution as "sex work"', *New Statesman* (1st December 2014). Also see Charlotte Shane against 'escort' and other euphemisms: 'Calling My Work What It Is', *Pacific Standard* (12th September 2015): https://psmag.com/economics/calling-my-work-what-it-is.

Jessie Sage, 'Does a sex worker's "sexual circuitry" get sunk by seas of sexual content?' (26th December 2019): https://www.pghcitypaper.com/pittsburgh/does-a-sex-workers-sexual-circuitry-get-sunk-by-seas-of-sexual-content/Content?oid=16399132. David is quoted in Michael Lambert's 'What Male Sex Workers Have to Say About Their Industry', out (10th August 2016): https://www.out.com/news-opinion/2016/8/10/what-male-sex-workers-have-say-about-their-industry.   Xoài Pham, 'Trans sex workers help people transform through intimacy', *We Are Your Voice* (3rd December 2019): https://wearyourvoicemag.com/lgbtq-identities/trans-sex-workers-transform-intimacy. Vince Ruston's excellent essay on the ambiguities of their former work: 'We Really Need You Tonight', *Kill Your Darlings* (4th September 2017):

https://www.killyourdarlings.com.au/article/we-really-need-you-tonight/.

On the dangers to doctors: A Vijendren, M Yung, J Sanchez, 'Occupational health issues amongst UK doctors: a literature review', *Occupational Medicine* 65 (2015), 519–28.

Sex Workers' Manifesto, First National Conference of Sex Workers in India (14th November 1997). Available here: https://www.nswp.org/sites/nswp.org/files/Sex%20 Workers%20Manifesto%20-%20Meeting%20in%20 India.pdf. Martha Nussbaum, '"Whether from Reason or Prejudice": Taking Money for Bodily Services', *The Journal of Legal Studies* 27 S2 (1998):, 693–723.

George Chauncey, *Gay New York: Gender, Urban Culture, and the Making of the Gay Male World, 1890– 1940* (Basic Books, 1994), especially the introduction. On the 'man's man' being defined against women, see Michael Kimmel's 'Masculinity as Homophobia', in *Privilege: A Reader* (Westview Press, 2003), edited by Abby Ferber and Michael Kimmel.

Karl Marx, *Capital*, Volume 1 (Progress Publishers, Moscow), translated by Samuel Moore and Edward Aveling. These Soviet printings of Marx are handsome and extraordinarily robust. My paperback edition of *The Economic and Philosophic Manuscripts of 1844* is not: International Publishers, 1969, translated by Martin Milligan.

Yolanda Estes's 'Prostitution: A Subjective Position' is from *The Philosophy of Sex: Contemporary Readings*; Melissa Petro, 'What being a Sex Worker Taught Me About Men', *Vice* (31st March 2018): https://www.vice. com/en_au/article/evqzq4/what-being-a-sex-worker-taught-me-about-men; 'Sophie' is quoted by Rose Troup

Buchanan in 'The Truth About Student Sex Workers: It's Far From Belle du Jour', *The Independent* (29th September 2014): https://www.independent.co.uk/life-style/health-and-families/features/the-truth-about-student-sex-workers-its-far-from-belle-du-jour-9757719.html. On protective cynicism among sex workers, see Ine Vanwesenbeeck, 'Burnout Among Female Indoor Sex Workers', *Archives of Sexual Behaviour* 34 6 (2005), 627–39.

Jeffrey Gauthier, 'Prostitution, Sexual Autonomy, and Sex Discrimination', *Hypatia* 26 1 (2011), 166–86.

On the personalities of johns: Melissa Farley, Jacqueline Golding, Emily Matthews, Neil Malamuth, Laura Jarrett, 'Comparing Sex Workers With Men Who Do Not Buy Sex: New Data on Prostitution and Trafficking', *Journal of Interpersonal Violence* 32 23 (2017), 3601–25. On punters being ordinary demographically: Philip Birch, *Why Men Buy Sex: Examining Sex Worker Clients* (Routledge, 2015).

Tilly Lawless's 'Gasp Under Gasp, Sigh Behind Sigh' is from *Doing It: Women Tell the Truth About Great Sex* (University of Queensland Press, 2016), edited by Karen Pickering.

On Venezuelan sex workers in Colombia: Michael Rummel, 'Some Venezuelan Refugees Resort to Sex Work in Colombia to Survive', *Voice of America* (4th February 2020): https://www.voanews.com/americas/some-venezuelan-refugees-resort-sex-work-colombia-survive. Martin Kyana spoke to Diana Wayonyi for '"The life I have lived has tortured me," says male sex worker in Mombasa', *DW* (18th June 2018): https://www.dw.com/en/the-life-i-have-lived-has-tortured-me-says-male-sex-worker-in-mombasa/a-44099058.

On transgender well-being in the United States: Christopher Carpenter and Gilbert Gonzalez, 'Transgender Americans are more likely to be unemployed and poor', *The Conversation* (13th February 2020): https://theconversation.com/transgender-americans-are-more-likely-to-be-unemployed-and-poor-127585. The quote about police violence against transgender sex workers is from: Kevin Nadal, Kristin Davidoff, Whitney Fuji-Doe, 'Transgender Women and the Sex Work Industry: Roots in Systemic, Institutional, and Interpersonal Discrimination', *Journal of Trauma & Disassociation* 15 (2014), 169–83. 'Billie' spoke to Kate Read in 'The Truth About Transgender Sex Work', *Popsugar* (19th March 2017): https://www.popsugar.com/love/Truth-About-Transgender-Sex-Work-43312813. Amber Ashton spoke to Allison Tierney for 'What Happens When Sex Workers Put Women of Color First', Vice (12th January 2018): https://www.vice.com/en_us/article/bjyp35/what-happens-when-sex-workers-put-women-of-color-first. On women of colour in the global sex work market, Kalama Kempadoo avoids paternalism and reductionism. See her 'Women of Colour and the Global Sex Trade: Transnational Feminist Perspectives', *Meridians* 1 2 (2001), 28–51.

Annie Sprinkle, 'We've Come a Long Way — And We're Exhausted!', in *Whores and Other Feminists* (Routledge, 1997), edited by Jill Nagle. The placard comes from Anna Tehabsim's 'Under red umbrellas, Germany's sex workers are fighting for fair treatment', Vice (5th March 2020): https://i-d.vice.com/en_uk/article/qjdeg5/international-sex-workers-rights-day-berlin-protest-law-change-prostschg-2020?Echobox=1583423869.

Amy Boyajian, 'Nobody Would Hire Me Because

I Was A Sex Worker. So I Started My Own Company', *Huffington Post* (28th November 2018): https://www. huffpost.com/entry/sex-worker-how-to-leave-industry_ n_5b463323e4b07aea7546b020. Andrea Werhun spoke to Graham Isador for 'Sex Workers Describe Their First Day on the Job', *Vice* (17th November 2016): https:// www.vice.com/en_au/article/7bm4za/we-asked-sex-workers-about-their-first-day-on-the-job. On prejudices among sex workers themselves: Lynzi Armstrong, 'Stigma, decriminalisation, and violence against street-based sex workers: Changing the narrative', *Sexualities* 22 7–8 (2019), 1288–1308. See also Tilly Lawless on homophobia among sex workers: 'Making space as a sex worker', *Archer* (16th January 2018): http://archermagazine.com. au/2018/01/tilly-lawless-making-space/.

Sarah Greenmore, 'I'm a sex worker in a legal brothel — here are the biggest misconceptions about what I do', the *Independent* (19th August 2015): https://www. independent.co.uk/voices/comment/im-a-sex-worker-in-a-legal-brothel-here-are-the-five-biggest-misconceptions-about-what-i-do-10460454.html. Lauren Rosewarne, 'Radical feminists' objection to sex work is profoundly un-feminist', *The Conversation* (8th August 2017): https://theconversation.com/radical-feminists-objection-to-sex-work-is-profoundly-un-feminist-81333.

On what men want from sex workers: Marian Pitts, Anthony Smith, Jeffrey Grierson, Mary O'Brien, Sebastian Mission, 'Who Pays for Sex and Why? An Analysis of Social and Motivational Factors Associated With Male Clients of Sex Workers', *Archives of Sexual Behaviour* 33 4 (2004), 353–8. Pitts and colleagues identify three factors, which they call 'Ease, Engagement, and Arousal'. On johns being well aware that sex workers might not be into them, see also 'Comparing Sex Workers with Men Who Do Not Buy Sex'.

Akiko's Boys

Taeko Kōno's 'Toddler-Hunting' is collected in *Toddler-Hunting and Other Stories* (WW Norton & Company, 2018, translated by Lucy North. I read the story in *Mānoa* 3 2 (1991), 42–57, by the same translator.

I am by no means a Kant scholar, but his notion of the apperceptive self thrills me. He discusses it in *Critique of Pure Reason* (Cambridge University Press, 1998), translated by Paul Geyer and Allen Wood. Robin Collingwood, *Principles of Art* (Oxford University Press, 1938). William James, *Psychology: The Briefer Course* (University of Notre Dame Press, 1961), edited by Gordon Allport.

John Williams on Kōno: 'Sex, Death and More Sex: Three Books of Fiction by Acclaimed Japanese Writers', *The New York Times* (January 11th, 2019).

On autopedophilia: Kevin Hsu and J. Michael Bailey, 'Autopedophilia: Erotic-Target Identity Inversions in Men Sexually Attracted to Children', *Psychological Science* 28 1 (2017), 115–23.

Julie Innes's definition of privacy is from the sixth chapter of *Privacy, Intimacy, and Isolation* (Oxford University Press, 1996). Gretchen Jones, 'Subversive Strategies: Masochism, Gender and Power in Kōno Taeko's "Toddler-Hunting"', *East Asia* 18 4, 79–107.

Jean-Jacques Rousseau's discussion of jerking off is from *Confessions* (Penguin, 1984), translated by JM Cohen. His *Reveries of a Solitary Walker* (Penguin, 2004), is translated by Peter France. I discuss the French philosopher's character and ideas (and botany) in *Philosophy in the Garden* (Scribe, 2019). Isaiah Berlin's *Freedom and its Betrayal: Six Enemies of Human Liberty* (Pimlico, 2003) has the title of a paranoid screed, but it is cautious and dignified. If anything, a warning against extremist politics of any stripe.

Susie Bright's 'Rape Scenes' is from *Sexual Reality* (Bright Stuff, 2008).

On the psychology of rape fantasies: Jenny Bivona, Joseph Critelli, and Michael Clark, 'Women's Rape Fantasies: An Empirical Evaluation of the Major Explanations', *Archives of Sexual Behaviour* 41 5 (2012), 1107–19; Susan Bond and Donald Mosher, 'Guided Imagery of Rape: Fantasy, Reality, and the Willing Victim Myth', *The Journal of Sex Research* 22 2 (1986), 162–83; also Leitenberg and Henning's 'Sexual Fantasy'.

Roxane Gay, *Hunger* (Corsair, 2018).

On moral looking, see Iris Murdoch's *The Sovereignty of Good*. Sigmund Freud's letter to Heinrich Gomperz is dated November 15th, 1899. It can be found in *Letters of Sigmund Freud, 1873–1939* (Dover, 1992), edited by Ernst Freud, translated by Tania and James Stern. Adam Philip's 'The Uses of Desire' is from *Side Effects* (Penguin, 2006).

Nancy Friday, *My Secret Garden* (Rosetta Books, 2013). On Friday's legacy (including its critics), see: Stephanie Theobald, 'Why Nancy Friday's 1970s collection of women's sexual fantasies still matters', the *Guardian* (November 6th, 2017); Anita Gates, 'Nancy Friday, 84, Best-Selling Student of Gender Politics, Dies', *The New York Times* (November 9th, 2017); Andi Zeisler, 'Friday's Children', *Bitch Media* (November 16th, 2017), available here: https://www.bitchmedia.

org/article/fridays-children/revisiting%E2%80%94and-
rethinking%E2%80%94-sex-positive-1970s.

John Dewey, *How We Think* (Dover, 1997).

Prince and Lady

Peter Webb's *The Erotic Arts* (Secker and Warburg, 1982) is a deep cache of joys, though his mistakes with this painting do give me pause. The painting itself can be seen here: http://collections.vam.ac.uk/item/O433068/painting-unknown/.

Sunil Khilnani's *Incarnations: A History of India in 50 Lives* (Penguin, 2017) is an excellent achievement. It makes a gargantuan history personal, without making it trite. Baden Henry Baden-Powell's note on Sansar Chand's collection is from his *Hand-book of the Manufactures & Arts of the Punjab* (Punjab Printing Company, 1872). Robert Aldrich's observation of British hypocrisy is from his 'Sex and Empire', in *The Encyclopedia of Empire* (John Wiley & Sons, 2016), editor-in-chief John McKenzie.

On Indian art and eroticism: MS Randhawa in *Kangra Paintings on Love* (Publications Division, Ministry of Information & Broadcasting, Government of India, 1962); Imma Ramos, '"Private Pleasures" of the Mughal Empire', *Art History* 37 3 (2014), 408–27. Richard Shusterman discusses ritualised sexual aesthetics in 'Asian Ars Erotica and the Question of Sexual Aesthetics', *The Journal of Aesthetics and Art Criticism* 65 1 (2007), 55–68.

Brihadaranyaka Upanishad, in *Upanishads* (Oxford University Press, 1998), translated by Patrick Olivelle.

On *tantra* in Hinduism and Buddhism: David White,

'Transformations in the Art of Love: Kāmakalā Practices in Hindu Tantric and Kaula Traditions', *History of Religions* 38 2 (1998), 172–98; Patton Burchett, 'Bitten By the Snake: Early Modern Devotional Critiques of Tantra-Mantra', *The Journal of Hindu Studies* 6 (2013), 1–20; Holly Gayley, 'Revisiting the "Secret Consort" (*gang yum*) in Tibetan Buddhism', *Religions* 9 6 (2018), 1–21; Amy Paris Langenberg, 'Sex and Sexuality in Buddhism: A Tetralemma', *Religion Compass* 9 9 (2015), 277–86; Paul Numrich, 'The Problem With Sex According to Buddhism', *Dialog* 48 1 (2009), 62–73. I include studies of Buddhism here because similar issues arise with *tantra*: the patriarchal exploitation of women and children, for example.

For an enthusiastic and handsomely illustrated (but far less critical) study of tantra, see Philip Rawson's *Tantra* (Thames & Hudson, 2012).

On *tantra* and the West: Sthaneshwar Timalsina, 'Encountering the Other: Tantra in the Cross-cultural Context', *The Journal of Hindu Studies* 4 (2011), 274–89. For an interesting discussion of Western feminists turning to Hindu ideas, see Brenda Dobia's 'Approaching the Hindu Goddess of Desire', *Feminist Theology* 16 1 (2007), 61–78.

On the *Kama Sutra* and sex in historical and modern India: Wendy Doniger, 'Reading the "Kamasutra": the strange & the familiar', *Daedalus* 136 2 (Spring 2007), 66–78; Wendy Doniger, 'From Kama to Karma: The Resurgence of Puritanism in Contemporary India', *Social Research* 78 1 (2011), 49–74; Jyoti Puri, 'Concerning *Kamasutras*: Challenging Narratives of History and Sexuality', *Signs* 27 3 (2002), 603–39.

Wendy Doniger, *The Hindus: An Alternative History* (Oxford University Press, 2009).

Some discussions of Hindu cosmology and its symbolism: Hans Penner, 'Cosmogony as Myth in the Vishnu Purāna', *History of Religions* 5 2 (1966), 283–99; Ankur Barua, 'Metaphors of Temporality: Revisiting the "Timeless Hinduism" versus "Historical Christianity" Antithesis', *Harvard Theological Review* 104 2 (2011), 147–69; Anannya Bohidar, 'Worshipping Breasts in the Maternal Landscape of India', *South Asian Studies* 31 2 (2015), 247–53.

Sigmund Freud, 'Symbolism in Dreams', in *A General Introduction to Psychoanalysis* (Liveright Publishing Corporation, 1935), translated by Joan Riviere. Also available electronically in a translation by Granville Stanley Hall. Sigmund Freud, 'Creative Writers and Day-Dreaming' in *Sigmund Freud: Art and Literature* (Penguin, 1990), translated by James Strachey.

Erich Fromm criticises Freud extensively in *Beyond the Chains of Illusion: My Encounter with Marx and Freud* (Continuum, 2009). He writes that the Austrian doctor's idea of universal mental health is 'actually the concept of a well-functioning member of the middle class at the beginning of the twentieth century, who is sexually and economically potent'.

David Cooper on the meaning of 'meaning': *A Philosophy of Gardens* (Oxford University Press, 2006). I wrote about Conan the Barbarian for *Island* 154 (2018). Clifford Geertz's nice line on culture is from 'Thick Description: Toward an Interpretive Theory of Culture', in *The Interpretation of Cultures: Selected Essays* (Basic Books, 1973).

The conversations between Martin Heidegger and Medard Boss are from *Zollikon Seminars* (Northwestern

University Press, 2001), edited by Medard Boss and translated by Franz Mayr and Richard Askay.

I am very wary of Richard Burton's 'translation' of *The Perfumed Garden of the Shaykh Nefwazi* (1886), but I believe the gist is clear enough in these passages. I could neither access nor afford a copy, but Jim Colville has translated the work more recently: *The Perfumed Garden of Sensual Delight* (Kegan Paul, 1999). Marisa Farrugia reviews Colville's translation favourably in *British Journal of Middle Eastern Studies* 32 1 (2005), 140–42. Farrugia also notes the original work's sexism.

On Schopenhauer: Bryan Magee, *The Philosophy of Schopenhauer* (Oxford University Press, 1997), especially 'Schopenhauer's Life as Background to His Work'; the sixth chapter of Peter Lewis's *Arthur Schopenhauer* (Reaktion Books, 2012); and Nigel Rogers and Mel Thompson's study of the 'rebarbative philosopher' in *Philosophers Behaving Badly* (Peter Owen Publishers, 2004).

Andrea Dworkin, *Intercourse* (Free Press, 1987). Martha Nussbaum, 'Objectification', *Philosophy and Public Affairs* 24 4 (1995), 249–91. On gender and feminism in colonial India: Padma Anagol, *The Emergence of Feminism in India*, 1850–1920 (Routledge, 2016); Padma Anagol, 'Agency, Periodisation and Change in the Gender and Women's History of Colonial India', *Gender and History* 20 3 (2008), 603–27; Durba Ghosh, 'Gender and Colonialism: Expansion or Marginalization?', *The Historical Journal* 47 3 (2004), 737–55, especially section V; Tanika Sarkar, 'Women in South Asia: The Raj and After', *History Today* 47 9 (1997).

Generous Promiscuity

Virginia Woolf, writing to Vita Sackville-West in December, 1928. From *The Letters of Virginia Woolf*, Volume 3 (Harcourt Brace Jovanovich, 1977), edited by Nigel Nicolson and Joanne Trautmann.

Acknowledgements

To my agents at Zeitgeist Media Group, Sharon Galant and Benython Oldfield: thank you, once again. You make the business of writing understandable and liveable.

I'm grateful to the gang at Scribe UK and Australia, with special thanks to: Philip Gwyn Jones for his tireless enthusiasm and editorial ambition; Sarah Braybrooke for her careful reading; Henry Rosenbloom for his unequivocal 'yes'; David Pearson for his striking cover; and Mick Pilkington, Kevin O'Brien, and Molly Slight for making all of this into an actual book. Thanks also to Francine Brody for her precise copy-editing.

I'm an Associate in the University of Melbourne's School of Historical and Philosophical Studies, and this position was enormously helpful for my research. Thanks to my colleagues there, and in the university library.

These scholars were generous with their expertise and research: Imma Ramos (British Museum), Brian Earp (University of Oxford), Matthew Looper (California State University), Cordelia Fine (University of Melbourne), Bree

Blakeman (Australian National University), Benjamin Hinson (Victoria & Albert Museum), Robert Aldrich (Sydney University), Greg Bailey (LaTrobe University), Danice Brown (Towson University), Michael Salter (University of New South Wales).

Thanks to Julie Koh and Yen-Rong Wong for their feedback on draft chapters, and to Kate Iselin and Corrine for hearing me out.

Amy Gray and others recommended erotic fiction: cheers, you shameless smut-peddlars.

To everyone I spoke to privately about your kinks: I'm chuffed by your trust and generosity. Keep doing what you're doing, mates.

My parents, Allana and David, encouraged me to treat sexuality with candour and honesty.

Apologies to Nikos and Sophia for being so embarrassing about this stuff. (Joke. I'm not at all sorry, kids.)

To Ruth Quibell, my love: thank you for your perseverance, generosity, and intelligence. I promise to never say '*yoni*' at you again.